TRIS

The Skinny, Sexy Mind

THE ULTIMATE FRENCH SECRET

DISCOVER HOW MASTERY OF THE ULTIMATE FRENCH SECRET
CAN TRANSFORM YOUR BODY AND YOUR LIFE.

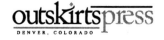
outskirtspress
DENVER, COLORADO

The Skinny, Sexy Mind
The Ultimate French Secret

Outskirts Press, Inc.
http://www.outskirtspress.com

ISBN: 978-1-4327-8862-9

Outskirts Press and the "OP" logo are trademarks belonging to Outskirts Press, Inc.

PRINTED IN THE UNITED STATES OF AMERICA

This book is dedicated to anyone who has ever felt like a prisoner in their own body, and especially to those who have mustered up the courage to pursue freedom in the skin they are in.

Thank you to my family and friends for inspiring me to become free and for encouraging me to share my joie and my message with others.

TABLE OF CONTENTS

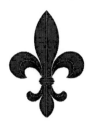

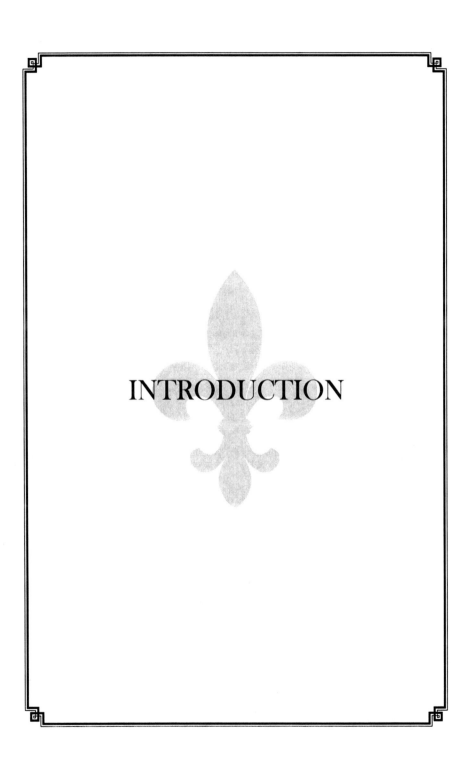

INTRODUCTION

INTRODUCTION

It has taken me twenty-six years to learn how to have a *skinny, sexy mind*. I have feared food and I have loved food; I have starved myself and I have gorged myself; and I have hated and tried to accept my body every step of the way.

Between the ages of 13 and 24, my existence was nothing more than seeking perfection in my body. I abused myself and trashed my body in this quest. Like a drug-addict, I had a secretive stash of laxatives, diet pills, and water pills, which became my primary sustenance. My life revolved around the daily effects that the pills had on my body and I became a master of excuses and explanations, so as not to blow my cover – that of a confident, well-adjusted student-athlete blessed with good looks and ready to claim the success that lay ahead. Exercise was the only drug that I didn't have to hide (quite the contrary): my six-hour workout sessions earned applause and emulation. As an elite athlete, it was easy to hide under the pretences of dedication and perfectionism.

My mind was like the Wall Street stock exchange boards, frantically performing calorie calculus and determining what effects the changes in numbers, whether up or down, might have. The mental anguish that imprisoned my mind is nearly impossible to describe. It is a prison of silence, humiliation, and desperation for self-acceptance.

Welcome to the minds of many American women – many more than you might think.

That silence is destroying the vitality of American women and children, and honest conversations about healing need to start now. We are a nation desperate for direction on how to live confidently in the present and in the bodies we are in. According to The National Institute of Mental Health, over eight million Americans – and one in ten women – live with a clinical eating disorder. A UNC Chapel Hill/SELF Magazine study revealed that 67% of American women between the ages of 25 and 45 struggle with disordered eating, which is any type of relationship with food that is abnormal or unhealthy. It has been reported in recent American surveys that 80% of ten-year old girls admit to following a self-prescribed diet and to fear of becoming fat. Despite our nation's obsession with diets and thinness, approximately two-thirds of American women are overweight or obese. We are a nation in a relentless quest for perfection in appearance and the thin ideal. Ironically if we can't be thin and perfect, we might as well be obese. We are Americans and we are extreme. We are a nation of people like me.

I found freedom and, more importantly, my voice, when I discovered France and *the* French secret in their *joie de vivre* lifestyle.

A Francophile turned Certified Personal Trainer and Lifestyle Fitness Coach, I have an affinity for French culture and the French approach to food, fitness, and body image. I spent two years as a curious American in France and attribute the experience to my own personal body image renaissance after my ten-year battle with eating disorders. *The Skinny, Sexy Mind* shares *the ultimate French secret* that changed my life and is transforming the lives of my clients. It is a path to self-discovery where you will learn to embrace every centimeter of your skin and find confidence in your body at last.

According to the U.S. Census Bureau's International Database on World Life Expectancy, the French are one of the healthiest, longest living people in the world. Many covet their *je ne sais quoi* mastery of confidence and their uncanny ability to eat, drink and be merry in health. The French legend of elegance never ceases to mesmerize and entice outsiders, most of whom are forever unable to pinpoint what exactly it is about the French that is so magnetic.

While Americans obsess relentlessly over working out, dieting, and plastic surgery in our efforts to be skinny, the French remain svelte and sexy, seemingly without effort. The concept of "fitness" in French doesn't even exist, and most Frenchmen could not be bothered with "working out" in the American sense. In fact, the words "fitness" and "workout" do not even translate into French – they are truly a foreign concept.

What does exist in France is a safely-guarded secret. It is a secret that is passed from generation to generation. It is the secret of living well in your skin. Knowing how to apply this secret to your life will empower you to stop personalizing the number on the scale and to actually start enjoying living.

I hope the ideas and experiences contained in this book will open your consciousness to this coveted concept that is deeply ingrained in the minds of young Frenchmen and Frenchwomen. It is simple and it is freeing: *être bien dans votre peau.* Translated literally, it means "to be well in one's skin."

This deceptively simple phrase *être bien dans votre peau* is the most widely used verbiage in colloquial French to describe someone with self-confidence and poise. In fact, there is no other translation for the adjective "confident" in the French language; this phrase conveys something better and richer than the English word "confident" can describe. The French are more than confident; they are *well* in their skin.

Together, we are about to begin a journey. The purpose of this journey is to learn how to master the art of living confidently in the truest way possible: from the inside out.

The French evoke mixed feelings for the average American. In many ways, Americans find themselves in a love/hate relationship with the French culture. The French woman is many American women's nightmare and dream. She is demurely sexy, effortlessly fit and stylish. She's intriguing, magnetic in love of life and beautiful. We want to learn her secrets, and want to be taught how to mimic her mysterious, irresistible sexiness. She is the friend we envy. We hate her because next to her, we feel frumpy and insecure. Not just that, even on our skinniest day, she makes us feel pudgy.

It is easy to be envious because we work hard and, in some cases, spend a fortune to get ourselves fit, and it comes so naturally to the French. It is as if they never even think about it; they just *are*. However, we *do* think about it – obsessively, in fact. Americans contribute to a multi-billion dollar weight loss industry that is growing exponentially every day. We pour our money into personal trainers, diets pills, cosmetic surgery, weight loss retreats, overpriced gym memberships and tasteless diet food. We think constantly about how we are going to lose weight and about what calorie-burning exercise we should be doing. We are engaged in an unending war-like relationship with the scale and merciless mirror.

What do the French do differently to be so beautiful and comfortable in their skin? Nothing. They do nothing. That's because "French fitness" is more than a lifestyle; it is a mindset. The reason the term fitness doesn't exist in the French vocabulary is because active living is a naturally ingrained aspect of their society.

Walk through the streets of Paris as an American, and yes, you will learn quickly that "direct" is a polite way to describe the French. Therefore, in an effort to be true *à la française*, I'll be direct as well: French "fitness" works because it is a lifestyle of moderation.

More than anything, theirs is a lifestyle of loving yourself. As you learn to love your skin, you will blossom into the most confident version of yourself you could imagine, and you will begin to learn what it means to be fully alive *à la française*.

I discovered the French secret six years ago while living and studying in Tours, France. During my second year living in France, I began to develop an analytic understanding of how the French, in embracing moderate hedonism, have mastered embracing life.

Living in the Dordogne region of southern France had always been a dream of mine; living alone, *sans* roommate, hadn't been part of the plan. Being alone had always translated into loneliness and nighttime binges for me – valleys of darkness that, for ten years, had plagued me in the form of yo-yo dieting, exercise bulimia, and concealed self-consciousness. In September 2006, I found myself on French soil and living alone in a small, semi-furnished apartment in the village of Périgueux, France. Against my will, I was confronting one of my greatest fears – being alone. Who would win the battle of darkness – food or me?

As a young American living in Europe, I worshiped my independence and emanated confidence. Deep inside, I was still victim to the vicious struggle of a distorted body image and my every move was controlled by food. How would I survive in a country whose streets permeate with the smell of freshly baked *pain au chocolates* and *croissants,* where "working out" isn't feminine, and where every other woman was genetically predisposed to be twenty pounds lighter than me?

Being in France was like being on Mars. All the dietary comforts that had armed me in my years of oscillating eating habits were non-existent. My mind was forced to transform. I had no choice. My sugar-free, fat-free, low-carb, high-protein, high-fiber, calorie-free foods weren't available. The local market taught me to savor full-bodied tastes: butter, *foie gras*, *chèvre* cheese, walnut bread, and red wine. The idea of restricting something from your diet is blasphemous to the French woman. Our American "all or nothing" mentality would be utterly bizarre to them. Moderation inevitably became my new foundation.

The common stereotype about the French was actually true: they don't get fat. Crazily enough neither did I. Even more strangely, this little blond American girl learned to mimic the French and their lifestyle secrets: guilt-free pleasures, moderation, and love for self. Over glasses of Bordeaux and Bergerac, hours of walking as a primary form of transportation, and endless dinner parties amongst French friends, I learned that I was beautiful.

A year later, I was a new woman. Périgueux, France taught me that balance isn't just a great idea, but an *attainable* way of living, *even in America*. This balance did more than bring stability to my health, eating and exercise; it freed me from years of addiction. French women, without saying one word, transformed my entire perspective on food, body image, and beauty.

This epiphany has been so powerful in my life that I have taken the power of its impact and transferred its message into my life mission and career. A certified personal trainer, certified lifestyle fitness coach and fitness entrepreneur, I am determined to share the Franco-American pathway to freedom with everyone I can. I am in the fitness industry to reach out to others who are stuck on the hamster wheel of body image discontentment and to embody a small piece of the *joie de vivre* that has enabled me to love my own skin.

I left France a beautiful woman; I came back to American *knowing* that I was a beautiful woman. Every woman in America deserves to know how to live confidently in her own skin and how to empower herself boldly, *knowing* that she is beautiful.

The journey begins here. Our first milestone in understanding ourselves is in understanding our relationship with food. As we begin our voyage, challenge yourself to be brutally honest and self-reflective, for that is that only way in which you will grow. Remember, there is nothing more invigorating than feeling free in your own skin and identity.

Let's begin! *On y va!*

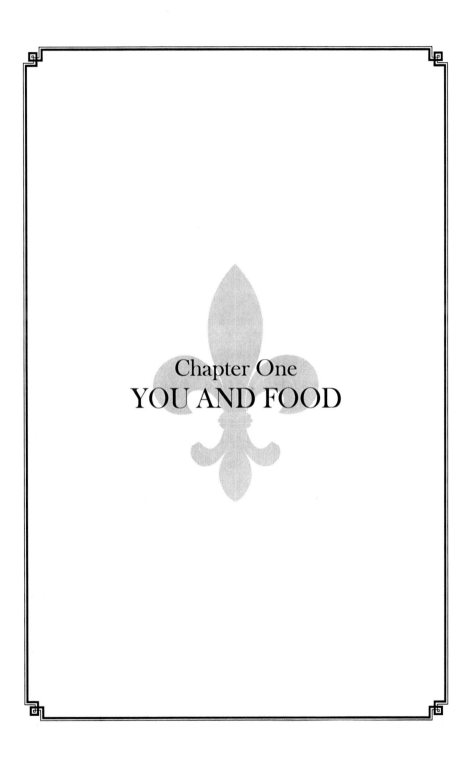

Chapter One
YOU AND FOOD

Chapter One
YOU AND FOOD

France worships food. Fine cuisine is admired and cultivated in the same way that we honor those in the NFL Hall of Fame.

From her earliest memory, a French youngster observes healthy interaction with food. The French child doesn't just eat or grab fast food from *MacDo*. No, the petite française *experiences* food. She savors the atmosphere and culture surrounding food. Her family nurtures this affinity in her, and she yearns to learn to cook.

She understands that to throw a proper dinner party, days of loving preparation are spent in the kitchen. Wine is chosen with precision and matched appropriately to each selected course. Guests arrive with cheer and vibrant table conversation, and debates unfold until the wee hours of the morning. The sharing of food fills the home with warmth, love, and a special ambiance. Even mundane errands for food are social for the French girl. She accompanies her mother daily to the local *boulangerie*, and understands that *croissants, pain aux noix* and the daily *baguette* come sprinkled with gentle gossip and tradition that infuses her daily life with a certain freshness.

While her French counterpart savors buttery indulgences with her mother, the average middle class American girl understands that attractive women resist bread, and most certainly avoid real butter. It is not explicitly told to her, but she is quick to understand what a refrigerator full of sugar-free jams and low-carb diet shakes means. The young American learns intuitively that "good living" is earned through control and self-discipline when it comes to food. The Française knows instinctively that her *joie de vivre* is founded upon her culture's appreciation for sharing food.

The average American child, grows up with few memories a dinner party or even a traditional daily family dinner. In 2006, *Time* magazine published an article entitled "The Magic of the Family Dinner." Researched by New York City's Colombia University's National Center on Addiction and Substance Abuse, the statistics that surfaced were alarming to say the least. On average, less than 47% of American families break bread together at least four times per week, and that percentage is diminishing rapidly.

America can't compete with France. The Centre National de la Researche Scientifique (le CNRS) released a scientific study in 2007 that revealed that approximately 84% of French families dine together "most (and/or) every day" of the week. French native Estelle Tracy summarizes the French perspective on this subject: "Family dinners are family binders."

Family dinners could be perhaps one of the single most influential factors in shaping a child's understanding of the role of food in his or her life.

Most Americans would recall their mother dieting during their childhood. Considering that 80% of American women are expressly dissatisfied with their appearance, we are a nation that is perpetually dieting. The Science Daily Editorial asserts that 75% of American women struggle with disordered eating, and an additional 67% of the remaining women are intentionally dieting. Without the support of these statistics, it would be impossible for the $50 billion dollar American diet industry to grow at the rate it does.

What is really happening here is that the American girl grows up watching her mother and role models demonstrate constant dissatisfaction with their bodies. They berate and belittle themselves, and experiment with every new Richard Simmons, Bow Flex, and Oxycise exercise tape on their inexorable quest to find contentment. Comparatively, a French girl celebrates the art of gastronomy side-by-side with her mother, sisters, cousins, and friends. She watches her mother embrace her sensuality in most everything she does, and learns how to keep herself active by strolling the promenade instead of punishing herself at the gym.

In my experience of growing up in America, I was raised to seek to understand the meaning of life and my purpose in it. I sought the ever-coveted "happy life" via the pathway of perfectionism. I wanted to be a perfect student and a perfect athlete, and have a perfect body. My body served as the singular means to an end; physical proof that I had achieved perfectionism in all of these areas. This was dangerous ground to tread, but it's a familiar theme in American culture. The happy life is the classic American Dream.

During my youth, I simply thought I was pursuing the American Dream and I felt a certain pressure to finish what my family started; the financial and time sacrifices that they made for my sports and my education made me feel incredibly indebted and fueled my need to excel. I believed everyone was living the American dream, so I began to pay close attention to people's actions and lifestyles in order to figure out what this idealized "happy life" really was anyway.

I watched my mother closely; I watched her fulfillment in teaching, coaching, and raising us diminished by the number that registered on the scale. Though my mother's greatest joy was based in being a mother and in her faith, I often watched her struggle to define her personal value and identity based upon the number that registered on the scale. I watched her because I wanted to mirror her and to understand what it was in life that was meant to make us happy and to give us purpose. I saw her punish herself with exercise and restrict herself from pleasurable foods. I was side-by-side with her every time she experimented with the newest diet trend, and I understood the respect she had for disciplined calorie consumption. Food was her enemy. The sole item hanging on our refrigerator door, attached with a magnet, was a piece of paper with her handwritten mantra: "Nothing tastes as good as skinny feels." My impressionable young mind instantly agreed.

Once the nest was finally empty, my mother committed more fully than ever to losing weight. She reconstructed her lifestyle by prioritizing exercise and adopting a no mercy approach toward counting calories. This discipline paid off and she lost fifty pounds but it meant that she and my father collided even more than ever over the issue of food and fitness. A pipefitter and steamfitter, my father still worked 14 hours days and spent another three hours a day in traffic to and from the construction site; he did not have the time, or admittedly the desire, to accompany her on this journey.

I was raised to believe that my father, clinically obese, didn't care enough about himself to properly take care of his health. My mother unknowingly instilled in me the idea that being fat was a disgrace, probably simply a reflection of her own inner fears and weight battle. Sadly, the truth is that my father, like many Americans, was over-committed and over-worked; his schedule barely permitted him time to spend both with his family and sleeping, so sleep usually became one of his last priorities. Sleep deprivation is one of the most influential factors in weight-gain and obesity, as the body needs a sufficient amount of sleep and rest to properly recover, rest and regenerate the body. Sleep deficiency not only sabotages the metabolism, but it often makes the deprived seek out energy from food with higher sugar or salt content to give them an immediate burst of needed alertness and energy. While Americans spend up to 60% of their income on mortgages and rent, Europeans spend a mere 15% on average. The difference between the two can all but sum up the difference in lifestyles. Americans buy bigger houses further away from the city where they work and spend most of their waking day either on the road back and forth to work or at work. Europeans live on a smaller budget, work less and can typically walk to work, permitting them more quality down-time with their family and friends and more hours to peruse the fresh fruit and vegetable *marchés* on a daily basis.

I grew up afraid of what food can do to one's body, and – as I naively believed – what it did to one's identity. During my entire childhood, I perceived my dad's identity to be tied directly to his weight. It wasn't until I was in college that I began to finally understand my father as a person; I was able to develop a more personal relationship with my father, independent of conflicts he had with my mom. My father has been overweight his whole life. After so many years of being teased, berated, and labeled as the "big, fat, funny guy," he has acquiesced in giving up on himself, too, and has lived emotionally protected behind his wall of largeness.

Not wanting to be negatively labeled by being even slightly overweight, I have spent my life making my body a machine. I wanted to be both the most elite of athletes and model-like skinny at the same time. What my body looked like determined what others would think of me. I was convinced that my body would influence my place in society.

While in France, my vision of the world and my body changed. Beauty, health, food and love, I discovered, are all ways in which to ascertain the meaning of living. This French mentality was my first experience of a liberated life promoted by good living rather than by success, money and materiality.

To understand the dichotomy between France and America I aim to highlight, let's conceptualize disordered eating and disordered body image. For starters, some facts: an eye-opening study conducted by UNC Chapel Hill and SELF Magazine recently reported that 75% of American women have some form of disordered eating, which is any type of relationship with food that is abnormal or unhealthy. That means that three out of every four women ages 25-45 struggles with disconnect between their body image (what they see in the mirror) and how that image affects their relationship with food. If you personally do not struggle with disordered eating, it is likely that someone you love does. It is a silently spreading sickness of alarming proportion.

The study also revealed that one in four women binge eat as a form of either self-sabotage, emotional release, or both. Binge eating, the consumption of large quantities of food in a short period of time, usually done in solitude, is currently a non-diagnosed eating disorder, falling under the category of Eating Disorder Not Otherwise Specified, or an EDNOS. From my own research in the health club industry and among college women, I can conjecture confidently that 95% of the women that do binge will never tell anyone about it. Binging is too humiliating and too sickening for the average woman to muster the courage to seek help. The woman that binges typically does it in the dark, in the car, or anywhere where she is alone. Post-binge, she battles a whirlwind of emotions: fear, guilt, humiliation, anger, and desperation.

Aside from the need to free these women's bodies from their prison of cyclical binging and purging, we need to reach out to our loved ones to free their minds from the mental anguish they fight. The typical woman who struggles with disordered eating allows her poor body image to consume her thoughts for over 50% of the day. Imagine what great things we will all be capable of once we free our minds from being enslaved to constantly thinking about ourselves, our bodies, or when our next meal is.

I speak from experience as a woman who has had food and body image control my thoughts for up to 80% of my day. When I was sick and deep in the darkness of my eating disorder, I was miserable, afraid and unable to share with anyone the extent to which fixating about calories, exercise and how my clothes fit not only consumed me, but controlled me. My happiness depended upon what the mirror told me, and the mirror could change its mind every hour depending upon which mirror I looked into. I feared using public restrooms because it meant I would encounter a potentially unfriendly mirror as I washed my hands. The anxiety of being disappointed in my image reflected in any given mirror even led me to washing up from an angle of the sink from which I would not have to see my reflection. I became scared of my own self. I was also nervous to shower, as the thought of seeing myself naked invoked great anxiety for me.

Confessing to someone and sharing the specifics of what true body image battling is was too intimidating and too humiliating for me to broach. I considered myself a generous, giving, loving person, but everything going on in my mind said otherwise; I was living contrary to the life of my mind. I was too disgusted with myself to admit to someone how insecure, selfish, and self-centered the majority of my thoughts were. I berated myself for allowing my life to be so disrupted because of a cause so superficial and empty. Admitting my need for help meant that I would have to admit I was a phony.

Body image disorders are no different than addictions. They must be identified and addressed, and a different, healthier lifestyle of living must be created. We must distract ourselves from past mindsets and guard our thoughts, for the mind is the wellspring of all living.

Disordered eating and EDNOS include: obsessive calorie counting, eating in secret, lifetime dieting, binging and purging, food addiction, emotional eating, and compulsive exercising. We are a nation of women who are fighting to disassociate guilt from food. We are so burdened by guilt (perhaps attributed to our puritanical roots) that we then intensify our focus on what image we believe we must look like. We are too hard on ourselves and we are too competitive with one another. Plagued by guilt of not measuring up or of over-indulging in something that is prohibited from our "diet" of thinness, we are a far cry from the liberal French (and European) hedonism that grants them the liberty to have a healthy association with body, mind, food, and spirit.

So there you have it – the American approach to self-evaluation: it is about achieving, perfection and beauty as status. France differs fundamentally from us in this area; there, life and appreciation of life is on a continuum, and each person's reality is uniquely beautiful.

While the French are notoriously xenophobic, they do manage to focus on their own self-development and personal expression more than their emphasis on others. As France's immigrant population continues to grow, the French *laissez-faire* attitude continues to develop and strengthen their ability to see pleasure and beauty in themselves and others.

French women master that *je ne sais quoi*, because, frankly, they don't give a damn about anyone else. Guilt is practically a foreign concept to the French. Rather than feeling guilty after over-indulging, the French take responsibility for and make modifications in their activity levels for a few days. In France, if something brings you and your body pleasure, indulge in it! The difference in such freedom of indulgence is that it removes the temptation to surpass the limit. The French are so detached from any semblance of food-associated guilt that they can actually partake in things in moderation; one piece of cake is a *petit plaisir*, not a black mark on a week of otherwise perfect dieting that becomes an excuse to finish off the entire cake. Moderation permits them then to properly savor and enjoy.

The ultimate difference between the French and Americans is that one culture focuses on understanding the meaning of living and the other the meaning of life. The choice is yours; the mindsets are entirely opposite. In America we are intently focused on *determining* the point of life, our place in it, and our identity in relation to our status in society

The French don't bother themselves with such ego-centric philosophy; if you don't understand life, well, "*c'est la vie.*" If you aren't sure of your place in life, figure out what little pleasures in life you do love and let those guide your daily life. Yes, the French will spend hours at a café philosophizing and churning over ideas of world politics and spiritual enlightenment; those are subjects of decorum, human growth, and intellectual honor. The French will not bother themselves obsessing over the personal lives of celebrities or over any other type of social status competitions. When the focus of your life is more directed towards impressing or competing with others, you have sacrificed your ability to live your own life. You are living for others rather than living for yourself.

The moment you stop living for yourself, you have shifted from *living life* to just trying to live. Every time you worry about how others perceive you, you have stopped living for yourself.

We tend to worry about what others think of us because, fundamentally, many of us lack the basic self-confidence that we need to flourish as human beings and live the life of joy that we were meant to live. By allowing others to define us based on their opinions and influences, we are not only running from our true selves but we are allowing others to define our existence. We need to know our true selves in order to break free from this natural tendency to allow others to define us. The happiest people in the world are those who know themselves and know what makes them happy; they exude confidence and dance like no one is watching.

Most people, regardless of gender, struggle with confidence. That means that every one of us is fighting to achieve that delicate balance of living for ourselves and not for others. When confidence is lacking, the root is either from having a too-obsessive focus on others' opinions or in an ignorance of one's true identity. A confident mind is unachievable without a deep grasp on what lies within the base of one's personality. It is impossible to be strong and confident if your focus is solely on other people's standard and perceptions.

Remember, the French have so mastered the concept of confidence that it is not even in the French vocabulary. If you want to refer to someone as being "confident" it is untranslatable. Instead, you describe them as *bien dans sa peau*, or well in their own skin. True confidence and joy go back to living fully and actively in the skin you are already in. It is impossible to achieve this if you don't love every inch and centimeter of skin on your body right now.

What I discovered in France made my vision and understanding of the so-called American Dream change forever. While my original

American Dream was founded on athletic success, goals for the future, and striving to be among the academic elite, my French-American Dream knew nothing of social praise or comparisons. My American Dream was nothing more than a measuring stick to prove my worth not only to myself, but to others. I was determined to prove that I was someone special, someone different, and someone worthy of being loved. I watched those who were successful in the States and mimicked their drive and determination, convincing myself that I was on the road to happiness. In all the different accomplishments I achieved on my journey – a National Age Group Record in swimming, the study-body presidency at my esteemed boarding school, a full scholarship to an academically prestigious college, academic awards and job promotions – I still always felt like I was missing the mark.

France inspired the right side of my brain. My left side, analytical and competitive, was abandoned, allowing my mind to be set free and to relish the carefree whimsy that comes in just living. Rather than continually trying to excel and be the best, I discovered that appreciation for beauty, health, food and love were all ways in which to discover the meaning of living.

Remember, it is your choice how you live and what you live for.

Confidence can begin to improve the minute you decide to improve the balance in your relationship with food. This starts by learning to celebrate food.

Lillian, my parents' plump, vivacious French neighbor recently brought over a bowl of *choux farcies* to comfort my mother after she had a rough day. Prepared specifically for my mom, this *lunch*, was delicately hand-prepared in the proper French style. Delivered to our front door in a glass bowl of broth, each little *chou* was carefully bound by a delicate chord, making them look like tiny parcel packages. Lillian had spent three hours soaking, unfolding and seasoning the cabbage.

She had laboriously diced onions, beef, turkey, and a kitchen-full of spices to create her masterpiece wrapped by the blankets of softened cabbage. She bounced through our front door, unannounced after a quick knock, declared proudly *"I's brought zou lunch girls,"* and an *"oh là itz hot!"* After proclaiming with some exasperation that she was exhausted, she refused any reciprocal hospitality and bounded back to her yard. Lillian loves to cook, and she loves to share her love.

Lillian has a healthy relationship with food and a firm understanding of the social network that is constructed around it. Lillian knows that food from a loving neighbor can not only provide health, but also comfort as a reminder that there is a neighbor that cares. The essence of food is that it celebrates community and connection.

We have a choice: celebrate food or fear it. For so many years of my life, I feared food. Lillian, like so many French women I know, makes me want to celebrate it.

America does celebrate food, but not with the gastronomical artistry that the French do. We celebrate it in unhealthy abundance. It is our filler and it is a cultural drug. It has set us up for a culture of dietary pitfalls that are affecting our physical health, mental health and life expectancy.

AMERICAN DIETARY PITFALLS

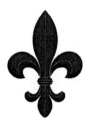

America is the land of abundance; the land of the obese. We are among those that make inappropriate and unapologetic assumptions about those who are overweight. Someone who is two hundred pounds overweight, must, we assume, overeat. We think that if they would just stop going to McDonalds and stop gorging themselves on Ben and Jerry's, then they would be a healthy weight.

Societal tendency is to judge and, unfortunately, we as individuals buy into that judgment. I cannot count the hundreds of people I have determined to be obese after performing a body composition analysis. Many of them are folks that come to me with a simple weight loss goal of ten pounds. They are shocked to learn the real state of their health and typically end up having an emotional breakdown. Obesity begins for women when their body fat percentage is 32% or higher, and for men when body fat percentage is 25% or higher. Ideal body fat is found in the range between 18-29% and 10-25% for women and men respectively.

America is so used to fat people that we cannot even distinguish obesity among ourselves. We are numb to what is healthy and what is not. This mentality is grounded in our habit of comparing and criticizing others. As America's waistlines have expanded, so has our definition of health. Since we are anesthetized to seeing a nation of morbidly obese, the reality of someone being fifty pounds overweight does not appear all that threatening by comparison. Take one short trip to Europe and you will be shockingly reminded of how far from health we have ventured.

Fundamentally, there are two issues at stake. One is that we are judgmental of others. The second is that we justify our own selves and worth based on comparisons to others. Insecure people judge others in order to build themselves up. *In comparing yourself to others, you will always lose in the end because you will never stop critiquing yourself.*

It is not our place to judge, especially not others' bodies. One common misconception about the obese is that they eat too much, but the truth is that not all fat people eat too much. In fact, most overweight Americans don't eat enough. This is a shocking statement to many people, but I see it again and again on a daily basis.

The majority of clients that approach me at the gym are starving for nutritional advice. They are desperate to know that their current diet will work, or that the magic weight loss pill they are taking is actually legitimate. Desperate for affirmation and results, many people stop eating.

Maybe they don't stop eating completely, but they take their caloric intake into dangerously low zones. Though it may seem counterintuitive, the body needs calories in order to burn calories. Too many crash dieters stop eating breakfast, eat only fat-free or extremely low-calorie synthetic foods and wonder why the weight doesn't come off as fast as they want.

Real weight loss, and by that I mean permanent weight loss and a healthy body weight, occurs through lifestyle changes and through the consumption of real food in moderation, not through dieting. The first thing I require of almost every client I have is to eat more food.

Over half of America skips breakfast and many people eat only once or twice a day. The body is meant to function at optimal levels of digestion and metabolic processing and the average American diet (along with the weight loss industry) is sabotaging our understanding of natural weight loss and health.

I use the French diet to explain moderation, balance and natural food to my weight loss clients. In order to move forward and to lose weight forever, they must understand that breakfast is the most essential meal of the day. Without breakfast you will never get your metabolism to the level of functioning at which it needs to be. Those who skip breakfast will be hungrier, moodier and less energetic throughout the day than will those who eat breakfast. Statistics have shown that non breakfast eaters tend to gain and hold weight more easily.

The body is meant to be fueled by food, so how can we expect to fill up our tank only partially and expect it to perform at optimal levels?

In this way, the body is like a car: if you try to drive your car without any gas, you will go nowhere.

The tragic thing about weight loss is that there are hundreds of thousands of Americans out there right now desperately trying to eat less to lose weight. The problem with extremely low-calorie diets is that the metabolic system – our engine for true calorie burning – goes into a catabolic state. In the catabolic state, the body thinks it is starving and in an effort for survival, it will hold on to any extra fat to keep the body warm and safe. Instead of using fat for energy, the catabolic body will begin to eat away at lean muscle tissue in order to compensate for the lack of fuel coming from food intake. When you destroy your lean muscle mass, you are destroying your metabolism and you are setting yourself up for a lifestyle of yo-yo dieting.

When there is an excessive calorie deficit, the body stores fat. Estrogen and cortisol levels skyrocket and the body holds onto problem area fat as it shuts down into famine mode. Estrogen, which is a female steroid hormone produced by the ovaries, contributes to the development and maintenance of feminine characteristics; when in excess, cortisol, an adrenal-cortex stress hormone, causes inflammation, irritation and a catabolic breakdown of lean muscle mass in the body, resulting in a decreased metabolic rate and ultimately fat storage.

Eating more when you are trying to lose weight can be a scary proposition. However, it is important to remember that it is all a matter of *what* you eat. You are what you eat, so choose to eat the right thing. Nationally renowned food-activist Michael Pollan summarizes every question about dieting and food with the following statement: "Eat real food." It can't be any simpler than that.

Choose to eat food that is fresh, in season, and locally grown. Pollan also advises that if it came through a window, it is not real food. If it is packaged and can sit on a shelf without decomposing, it is not food.

I challenge you to take a risk here. Do something that is counterintuitive to your years of dieting, and eat MORE. You have nothing to lose and everything to gain here. I encourage you to make an appointment with a dietician or certified nutritionist to get your resting metabolic rate (RMR) tested. This will give you pointed direction to the amount of calories your body needs for survival. You should never drop below your RMR when trying to lose weight.

It is important to distinguish between a lofty desire and a legitimate goal. The only way to achieving your body's natural, healthy body weight is by reconstructing the way you eat. It takes about three weeks for your taste buds to change, and once they do, I promise you will never want to go back to sodium-loaded, processed substitutes for food again. Your entire relationship with food will change and you will start to see food as both nourishment and pleasure. Since you will be fueling your body consistently throughout the day and since nothing will be off limits, your struggle with over-eating and over-indulging will likely be a thing of the past. Over time, with proper activity levels, your body shape will morph naturally and more effortlessly than you expect.

I fought for years and years to accept myself. I starved myself for the good part of my high school and college years, afraid to eat most foods. As a trainer who has finally learned the science behind nutrition, I've realized that it's not a gamble; it's a science. To lose fat, you must have muscle mass because muscle burns fat. To have muscle, you must workout and correctly train your muscles to force growth. To maintain muscle, you must eat. And I mean eat.

My clients who struggle with weight loss are the stubborn ones who refuse to eat as I have guided them. When they consume less than 1200 calories per day, their bodies go into famine mode and an onslaught of hormonal changes ensues, which, drastically slows their metabolisms. Fluctuations of the metabolism not only influence weight gain or loss, but affect general long-term functionality of the thyroid. Moreover, most dieters have high levels of stress associated with their diet and desire to lose weight. Increased stress levels and lack of sleep impair the body's ability to function. Stress causes the hormone cortisol to increase in the body, and cortisol puts on belly fat. In order words, starving dieters are sabotaging themselves in the short-term *and* long-term, and the more they stress about it the fewer results they will see.

Go natural, and life becomes much easier. Listen to your body and feed it well, and it will find its own rhythm. When you are no longer consumed or confused by the food you should or shouldn't be eating, you will find that you have a whole lot more time and freedom to actually enjoy living.

Low calorie intake is an all too often an overlooked culprit in the sabotage of weight loss goals. Extreme calorie restriction deprives your body of nutrients and energy, making it difficult for your body to obtain sufficient energy for vital functions. When protein intake is insufficient, the body finds protein from other areas, such as blood, the liver, and tissues to break down for energy. If someone is trying to lose weight over an extended period of time by eating fewer than 1,200 calories or less than their RMR, their bodies break down muscle tissues instead of fat for the needed energy. Low calorie intake paired with extreme exercise is a recipe for disaster.

When an individual with a too-low caloric intake partakes in heavy training sessions, he/she undergoes gluconeogenesis, where glucose is produced from non-carbohydrate supplies, typically from the amino acids found in protein. Therefore, instead of losing body fat mass, these individuals lose lean muscle weight by allowing the components that already exist in their muscle tissue to be broken down. Low-calorie dieters suffer from similar side effects as those suffering from ketosis: headaches, bad breath, dizziness, chronic fatigue, and nausea. Workout expenditure is very difficult, and time at the gym is handicapped due to a basic lack of energy.

Anyone on low-calorie diets will not hold up well to the training necessary to achieve optimal fitness and overall health and well being. Being depleted of energy and suffering from bothersome side effects of insufficient calories, these 1200-calorie dieters will have a difficult time maintaining their eating habits. Since a high percentage of weight loss comes from muscle mass and water weight, dieters typically put any weight lost right back on after finishing the diet. It is not a realistic or a healthy way to build a lifestyle. Extreme fatigue also makes it difficult for this diet to provide long-lasting results, as it becomes more and more difficult and exhausting for the dieter to maintain such a lifestyle.

I have since doubled my calorie intake from what it was during my dark years of calorie restriction and over-exercising, and, as a result, my weight and body fat have dropped. Keep in mind that, due to my athletic training in my adolescence, I was typically working out four to five hours per day between the ages of 14 and 24.

I was the athlete that did everything a coach asked and more. I secretly added workouts that no one knew about, I did extra cross-training, and I thought constantly about how many calories every workout burnt. Not only was I overtraining, but I was under-eating.

I was an extreme example of many gym-goers I see today. Back then, I ate approximately 1200 to 1500 calories daily, usually distributed amongst two to three meals. After I got tested and learned that my resting metabolic rate was over 1900 calories, I began consuming 2400 – 2800 calories, eating six to seven times a day. On days that I worked out more than usual, my caloric intake increase over 3,000 calories.

I am leaner, stronger and more toned than I have ever been in my life. I eat double what I used to and I work out less. I've learned the hard way, through years of trial and error, that it really is about science and going back to what is natural for the body.

Before I became a trainer, I fled from carbohydrates, ate fat-free everything, and barely got 50 grams of protein per day. I drank more Diet Coke than water and I slept five hours a night. Who would have thought that by eating more (consistently) that my body would finally look the way I have always wanted? That suddenly, *I* would be the chick in the gym that women went to for advice?!

Training five hours a day is now out of the question, because it's counterproductive. Overtraining and under-feeding your body is a double-whammy combo that does absolutely nothing for you aside from eating away at your lean muscle mass and subsequently slowing down your metabolism. I currently max out my training at two hours per day, and most days it's only an hour to an hour and a half. The exception to that rule is if I am training for a marathon or long triathlon, necessitating a longer, endurance specific workout. I determine my training schedule by listening to my body. We cannot allow ourselves to forget that the body is a marvelous – and smart – machine, if you learn to listen to it properly.

It is painful to watch so many like me slave away and narcissistically force themselves into the cycle I call "starve, sweat and stay the same." It hurts me so much because I've been there and suffered through it. Life is too short to be lived like that! For me to discover this truth, I first had to discover France. France permitted me to realize that life is meant to be better and that food is meant to be enjoyed guiltlessly. I much prefer the French attitude and I implore each one of you to find a way to change your relationship with food.

You may be wondering how to begin to change your relationship with food and learn to eat, drink and be healthy. It is simple really, and begins with knowing what you put into your body and your reaction to that fuel. This can be accomplished by keeping a food journal.

The key to changing your view and understanding of the role of food in your life is in keeping a proper food journal. You will write down not only everything you eat or drink, but also what time you consume it, your emotional mood, and the nutritional facts about the product itself. If you do not know *exactly* what you are fueling your body with, then you will never *exactly* achieve your fitness goals. Most people have no idea of what they actually consume per day, and when it comes to being healthy and losing weight, it ultimately comes down to simple math: calories-in versus calories-out.

Your first week of journaling will be about educating yourself. Label-reading will be tedious at first, but will soon become natural and quick once you know exactly what you are looking for and what to avoid. Start to create the habit of recording your thoughts as soon as you eat something. This requires discipline. If you truly want to achieve your goal, you must have discipline. A lot of people complain that they are too lazy to stay consistent with food and journaling; you are only too lazy if you choose to be. Change has to matter to you in order to care enough to make an effort. Every day you will have a choice: be disciplined or be lazy.

Your first week you will keep track of food and drink consumed: the time, the portion size, and the number of calories. Also, at the bottom of each entry, calculate your daily calorie totals and track your physical activity levels.

After the three weeks of journaling, you have now created a habit.

Knowledge is power; you need to know what is in everything! Keep in mind, though, that knowing does NOT mean obsessing. The goal is to ultimately not need to journal, but to develop a pattern of healthy food intake as a lifestyle.

The key to success in eating is *moderation*. I have never told a client to diet. You should see the relief that comes across people's faces when I free them from the concept of dieting. In my opinion, one should avoid anything in life that begins with the word "die." We're talking more about positive lifestyle change, and one that can be very different from America's current lifestyle. It will take a little more preparation and planning, but these small acts will go a long way. Nothing is off-limits, but you must know that some choices have consequences. This is where journaling about your emotional state will be useful. If you don't take the time to slow down and consider how a certain food makes you feel both physically and emotionally, then you will never know how to develop and change your entire relationship with food. If there is something that you eat that causes you guilt, you need to analyze why and find a way to balance that guilt with moderate consumption.

For many people, food can be a drug. We are a society that has a tendency toward addiction and we are surrounded by advertisements for food everywhere we turn. We are addicted to the feeling of full bellies, deliciously greasy fare, and having food dictate our daily lives. The marketing of most food promises us happiness with consumption, and we all too happily give in.

The question that the individual truly wanting change must ask is whether or not they live to eat or eat to live. When you consider that 45% of American adults are obese, and – an even more staggering thought – that 50% of our children are extremely overweight, then it becomes clear that we are a society that is divided in a myriad of ways.

We are at war with ourselves. We are at war for survival. Food is drugging our children, our future generations, and the life expectancy of our parents. Every year in America there is an increase of money spent to educate on health, nutrition, the obesity epidemic, and on fitness, however, ironically, the rate of obesity is only increasing despite our efforts to change and educate. For many people, especially middle to low-income families, the cost of nutritious food is unconceivable for their budget. The cheapest way to feed a family in America is through processed, frozen or fast food. It is no wonder that higher obesity rates are linked with low-income and minority families; with the industrialization of food and outrageous cost of healthy, organic choices, we are dooming people to a fate of fatness before they even have a fighting chance.

The average European's day revolves around food, but in a very different, more enlightened way. The typical Parisian purchases groceries every day, whether from the *supermarché*, the corner *charcuterie* or the *boulangerie*. They insist on fresh food and since the nation hasn't entirely industrialized food processing the way we have in the States, they tend to buy and eat only what is locally grown and produced. The idea of "organic" often doesn't even exist in Europe because everything is automatically organic.

Shopping for food is actually a social event, and the planning of the menu becomes more of an art than a formula for consumption. The American soccer-mom would argue that such a leisurely lifestyle just isn't realistic, that making it to Costco once a week for a family shop-up is demanding enough. Now throw in working, picking up and dropping off kids at various events, commuting, working out at the gym and (God forbid) actually cooking dinner.It is understandable why pizza delivery, ordering-in, and drive-thrus are the crux of our alimentary base. They are God-sends in the name of convenience for the over-worked, over-scheduled American family.

France revolves around food, but the French don't. How is that possible? France is rich in gastronomic history, agricultural cultivation, and regional pride. The sun rises on cobblestone streets wrapped in the sweet warm smells of fresh baking bread, and it sets upon the bitter aromas of aged wine being shared among friends during six course dinners on Tuesday nights. Cheese makers are revered for their master craftsmanship, and everyone in town knows their daily *pain au chocolat* is a healthy necessity.

The French *appreciate* food. They savor it, they see beauty in it. Never would they abuse it or feel that they need to over consume a specific food because it is a splurge. Food is the essence of their social lives because they take much joy and pleasure in sharing, discovering, and comparing tastes.

The majority of Americans are either afraid of food or addicted to it. We need to reconcile these extremes in order to be free to celebrate the joy that food can bring to our lives and to our self-awareness. It's time to start tasting food *à la française* and to start experiencing it rather than just consuming it.

To begin, always inhale deeply through your nostrils when entering a kitchen, when cooking, when being seated at a restaurant, and right when your plate is served to you. Next, cleanse you palate. Drink enough water to not risk being thirsty during your meal, and so that you can fully taste every flavor and spice of what you are about to eat. Take a bite, a small one. Cut your food into smaller portions than you would normally. You have to remember that, if you have lived in America for a long period of time, chances are that your understanding of bite-size and portion-size is extremely inaccurate and warped. Now, chew slowly. Allow the food to flood your entire mouth taste it on your tongue, on the roof of your mouth, and as it begins to journey towards your throat. Food should be chewed 10-25 times before being swallowed. Every three bites or so, sip more water, re-cleanse your palate, taste something new, and compare tastes.

At a renowned bakery in Tours, France I had the opportunity to attend a four-hour seminar on proper tasting and the use of taste buds in wine and cheese combinations. The baker insisted that we incorporate every sense and space in our mouth to engage the full flavoring of what we were eating. He jumped passionately from person to person, leaning down to our faces to be able to smell the combos of bread, cheese and wine we were constructing on our own as we brought them to our mouths. This monsieur was a true artist. He wasn't just instructing us in how to appreciate a proper French wine and cheese tasting; he was sharing an art. The beauty and creativity he expressed in describing the different possible tastes, textures, combinations, smells and origins of the wine, bread, cheese and olive oil made me realize that this wasn't merely a tasting or a glimpse into French tradition – this was a rebirth of art in my soul.

This was the beginning of my awakening that food could have a different role in my life than what I learned in America. I was hungry to master my new understanding and budding relationship with food.

Before that moment in Tours, food was an unpredictable enemy. I never knew how it would affect me and whether or not I could control my portions. I never felt satisfied or at peace with anything I ate, and my concern about caloric intake dominated any consumption I would have enjoyed. The moment my stomach was uncomfortably full, my self-esteem plummeted. I would chide myself for my poor decisions and lack of control. I distorted images of myself in my head and envisioned myself as noticeably ten to fifteen pounds heavier.

Then I would binge. Well, I'd rather call it overeat, but in truth it was a binge. Food became my drug, as it is for many Americans. When stressed, bored, or anxious, I would eat till I was numb. It was a way to emotionally distract and numb myself from what was really bothering me. I ate until I was so disgusted at my full, bloated, upset stomach that I would swear to never eat again. To off-set these binges, I would skip breakfast, take laxatives, overdose on thermogenic fat burners and force myself to throw up. During high school, I used to over-exercise to purge the excess calories from my secret binges. Something sadistic in me liked the excruciating stomach aches I got from my Ex-lax overdoses and the muscle pain I would get from my exhausting workouts; it was like self-inflicted punishment.

This compulsion, when the end of the purge finally came, would bring cathartic enlightenment. It was as if, after gorging myself on as much food possible, I could prove to myself that food is not the answer to life, because see my problems were still there no matter how much food I ate. Strangely enough, it felt philosophical to discover that, after an hour of self-abusive behavior and a humiliating weakness, I was still me. The pain of it all made me feel fully alive; since my understanding of living was limited, I needed to feel deep suffering in order to appreciate true elation again.

Unfortunately, I am not alone in the self-sabotage cycle. Thankfully, the *skinny mind* and *joie de vivre* that I discovered in France saved me.

Writers John and Stasi Eldredge poignantly explain the ache I felt in their book *Captivating*:

When it comes to the issues surrounding beauty, we [women] vacillate between striving and resignation. New diets, new outfits, new hair color. Work out; work on your life; try this discipline or that new program for self-improvement. Oh, forget it, who cares anyway? Put up a shield and get on with life. Hide. Hide in busyness; hide in activities; hide in depression. There is nothing captivating about me.

We find ways to numb ourselves. We are afraid of our own beauty; we know that it's there and we know that it is the essence of who we are, yet we fear ourselves. We know that there is power in our beauty, but we fear amounting to being nothing more than a disappointment and a washout. It's like watching a former beauty queen who has been tarnished by the weight of the world; she walks around in sad resignation of the beauty that formerly identified her. Deep inside all of us lies the terrifying thought that we are just fighting to maintain a façade of what and who we thought we were. We are terrified that whatever truly defined the beauty of our youth is impossible for us to maintain for life.

In her book *A Return to Love: Reflections on the Principles of a Course in Miracles*, Marianne Williamson captures the essence of beauty that we are all desperate to understand about ourselves.

Our deepest fear is not that we are inadequate. Our deepest fear is that we are powerful beyond measure. It is our light, not our darkness that most frightens us. We ask ourselves, Who am I to be brilliant, gorgeous, talented, fabulous? Actually, who are you *not* to be? You are a child of God. Your playing small does not serve the world. There is nothing enlightened about shrinking so that other people won't feel insecure around you. We are all meant to shine, as children do. We were born to make manifest the glory of God that is within us. It's not just in some of us; it's in everyone. And as we let our own light shine, we unconsciously give other people permission to do the same. As we are liberated from our own fear, our presence automatically liberates others.

This is why beauty is so powerful. It is important that we understand that it is OK to embrace our beauty. How does it cause women to ache so desperately, young girls to starve themselves so and grown women to give up on life? Eldredge explains the essence of beauty's power: "Beauty *nourishes*. Beauty *comforts*. Beauty *inspires*. Beauty is *transcendent*. Beauty says, *All shall be well*." It is no wonder we are so obsessed. Doesn't everyone simply want to know fundamentally that all shall be well? True beauty is beauty that invites the beholder to rest.

That fundamental concept of rest is, in my opinion, exactly what makes the French so distinctively and so beautifully French. French women are at peace with food, and they are at peace with their bodies. It is a restful system of wellness, a sort of give-and-take of life and appreciation for the beauty of small things. They are a nation that believes in vacation, where the average employee receives a minimum of five weeks paid vacation per year, and between those five weeks and French national holidays, most French workers are off for up to 39 days per year. In America, you are blessed if you have a job that allows you with one week of vacation. The implications of such a difference make a tremendous impact on society and on an individual's ability to rest, slow down her pace of life, and smell the roses.

I learned from the French that it is a system of checks and balances. After nights when my allotted glass of red wine turn into three or four, I now instinctively find myself on the treadmill early the next morning. Please note: I am not speaking of punishment like binging and purging, as in my former days. Rather, it is a system of balances, when a *petit plaisir* turns into a splurge, I want to reverse it and sweat out the toxins. I have incorporated this French system of balances and it has helped me create a reaction of moderation, and of give-and-take, when something in my diet becomes out of whack. When I finish such a moderate, make-up workout, I feel unbelievably cleansed, relieved, and detoxified. When I re-achieve my natural state of balance, I feel alive again.

The French live similarly; it is an approach of well-being or *bien-etre*. I remember well one night of debauchery with my French co-worker Sébastian. The night of extravagance in Bordeaux ended around four in the morning, and only a few hours later, Séb was up for a waterside walk to cleanse his body before a breakfast of freshly caught oysters and chilled chardonnay.

The French love food because they know how to savor and appreciate it. Simply put, they know how to eat for pleasure. They eat just enough to enjoy the decadence of what is in their mouth, and know that they don't need to over-indulge, because, well, they can eat it again anytime they want. This cultivation in appreciation for tastes, textures and sensory awareness is a lifelong journey. The ability to eat and drink for pleasure comes in the ability to savor small portions. For example, I have a much more refined appreciation for the tannins and distinct taste of a Bordeaux in my first glass of wine for the night than I ever will have on my fourth. The fourth glass therefore, (and possibly the third and second as well) is an utter waste.

When you rid yourself of the deprivation mentality that comes with dieting, it is easier to stay within the parameters of portion control. Loved your glass of wine tonight? Great, have another tomorrow. Did that *chocolate chaud* satisfy your most desperate hormonal craving? Fantastic, permit yourself to innocently indulge tomorrow, as well, if you so wish.

The most general guideline I can give for when it comes to listening to your body is simple: eat for pleasure. Many would say that that is what we do as Americans, right? Yes, we do, but it depends upon how you define pleasure. Is it pleasurable to eat while driving? If you are driving and watching the road, are you able to focus on the complex taste combinations of a food and really enjoy the sensation of eating it? Is it pleasurable eating past comfort level at a restaurant or at all-you-can-eat buffet because you want to get your money's worth? Do you really taste and appreciate the delicacy of food if you are eating in front of the television, numb to the process of eating itself?

True culinary pleasure should be an exquisite, complex art. Food is a textured cloth that interweaves family and friends and creates the pillars of social exchange. Eating is needed nourishment to the body and soul; it is a beautiful concept celebrated since the beginning of time.

Families that break bread together stay together. Lovers get to know one-another over tables of food where opinions are exchanged and tastes are developed and discovered. Food is not only a form of sharing and communion, but also of self-discovery.

Find what it means for you to develop a pleasurable appreciation for food. If you instinctively answer: "because it tastes good," then, my friend, you are at a remedial level…but there is still hope! Identify the textures; ask yourself *why* you like what you like. Is it food association that you value? Or perhaps it is the textures of food that you prefer? What memories do specific foods bring to mind? What it is about flavor that stands out to you? Force yourself to identify specific words of description for the taste, texture, presentation, and memory association of everything you flavor.

FRENCH EATING GUIDELINES

- Eat for pleasure

- Eat until you are no longer hungry

- Never allow yourself to feel full

- Look at your food and enjoy the presentation of the dish

- Eat every three hours

- Eat real food; food that is fresh and local

- Flee from processed foods and additives you cannot pronounce

- Fast food must be consumed at an absolute minimum, if at all

- Drink 0.75% of your body weight in ounces in water daily

- Make food journaling a habit

- Cheating on nutrition is only cheating yourself out of results

Real lifestyle changes start in the heart and mind. You have to start loving yourself and getting to know yourself in order to start liking you. Once you like yourself, it is much easier to stay committed to dietary changes or a workout routine. As your mind changes and you start to love the skin you are in, your *skinny mind* will allow you to grow in self-respect and ultimately self-confidence, and the weight will fall off of you.

Success in health and fitness is attained solely through a balanced approach to food and nutrition. America must break the cycle of making food our goal. We must stop rewarding our children with treats to eat. Our nation is teetering between obesity and eating disorders and we wonder why we are so plagued by these diseases compared to the rest of the world. Our state of health is a direct reflection of our own warped perception of food.

YOU AND FOOD.
Skinny, Sexy *à la carte*

Un jour sans vi nest comme un jour sans soleil.
[A day without wine is a like a day without sunshine.]

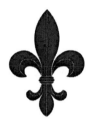

i. Skinny, Sexy SUMMARY:

Our first milestone in understanding ourselves is understanding our relationship with food. The French appreciate food, savor it, and celebrate it. Food should be a pleasurable part of life.

ii. Skinny, Sexy REFLECTION:

How does food influence your mood on a daily basis? *Do you feel like your life has been a constant diet, or do you not permit yourself to eat some things?* Do you often feel guilty after eating? *How many times a day do you think about food?* How does what you eat or don't eat affect how you see yourself in the mirror?

iii. Skinny, Sexy PRACTICAL APPLICATION:

Spend a week trying to evaluate what foods bring you most pleasure. Slow down when you eat this week. Try to engage all senses of pleasure while eating so that you not only taste, but start to savor these foods. Do not outlaw any foods this week and do not eat diet food; eat in frequent, small portions and see if your attitude towards food changes. Remember, nothing is off limits; everything is allowed in moderation.

iv. Skinny, Sexy EATING:

Start writing down what you eat; track what it is, what portion size you are eating, what time of day it is, and how you feel after eating.

v. Skinny, Sexy YOU:

It's time to start owning your own beauty. Owning your own beauty is rooted in confidence. If you don't feel confident, fake it until you make it. Eventually your mind will start believing it. Start this self-acceptance by looking into a full-length mirror for ten minutes. Compliment yourself as much as you can and stop yourself every time you say something negative. At the end of the session, write your list down somewhere you can easily refer to later.

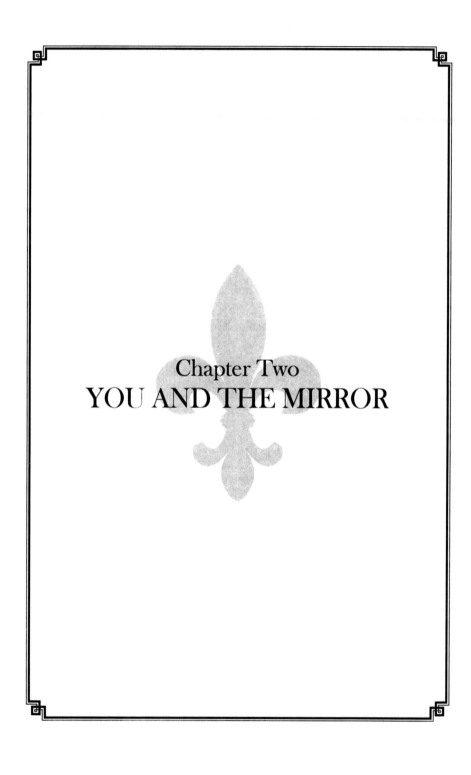

Chapter Two
YOU AND THE MIRROR

Chapter Two
YOU AND THE MIRROR

The mirror is an ironic thing. We are enticed by the drawing power of its reflection and we empower it with the authority of a judge in a courtroom, allowing it to determine a verdict of our worth, beauty, and identity. Self-recognition through reflected images is one of the innate qualities that make human beings capable of empathy, self-awareness, and advanced social abilities. It is only natural that, from an early age, we are drawn to mirrors.

Unfortunately, for many of us at some point in our lives, the image in the mirror begins to betray us. Author Regina Franklin describes this infidelity of image recognition in her book *Who Calls me Beautiful?* She explains the unpredictability of the mirror in her daily life:

> I cannot remember the exact day the mirror became my prison, but I knew I was being held against my will when I realized I was seeking affirmation from an object that could only reflect what I chose to see. Certainly there were some days when I walked away from my morning mirror routine thinking, "Not too bad." But more often were the "if only" days. "If only my hair where longer." "If only my hair

were shorter." "If only I were taller." "If only my eyes were brown." And the ever present "If only I were thinner."

Everyone has a relationship with the mirror to some extent. How would you describe yours? The seeds of disordered eating and distorted body image sprout from the reflection you see in the mirror, so it is important that you understand how it is involved in your daily life and the impact it can have on your mind.

We often mistakenly presume that eating disorders are things found among teenagers and women only. The battle for body image begins at all ages and affects both sexes. Approximately 1 million American men struggle with an eating disorder. Men make up an estimated 10% of those with anorexia and bulimia, and up to 35% of those with binge eating disorder. Some who battle with the mirror are children, others are in college, and even more are adults.

My distorted body image developed at the young age of 10. As a young girl, I worshipped my mother; she was my best friend, my confidant, and my teacher (literally; I was home-schooled). She was loving and beautiful, but I could tell she harbored disappointment in herself. I always knew my mother loved me unconditionally, but she was not one to lavish words of praise on a daily basis, since she did not experience that as a child either. I remember, however the most sought form of praise in our house was for athletics – so excel in athletics I would. When I broke the National Age Group Record in the 100 yard Freestyle I discovered how addicting the praise of others felt and I began to value what others thought of me. All the while, it was beyond my ability to comprehend why my beautiful mother was perpetually dieting and so dissatisfied with herself. All the calorie counting she engaged in, all the trendy diets, and all the trips to the gym opened my eyes to the relationship of fear and respect my mother had with food.

At age 12, I hit a plateau athletically and immediately attributed my lack of improvement to my maturing body. This is a common in the sport of swimming, as swimmers practice and compete in skin tight Lycra; the more hydrodynamic you are in the water, the faster you will swim. The changes in my body made me panic and so I mimicked any diet trend that I came across. Moreover, the issue of weight often came up in family arguments and, as an adolescent who did not understand the complicated roots of these conflicts, I associated thinness with love.

I began to diet. I lamented to my journal, "113 lbs, need to be under 110, *soon.*" I started staring at my image in the mirror and thinking in terms of *if only's*. *If only* I was skinnier, then I would be faster in the water. *If only* I was thinner, then maybe my family wouldn't fight so much. *If only* my hair was longer, then I would get more attention from the boys I liked.

My entire memory of my elite boarding school experience in high school revolved around *if onlys* and calorie counting. I no longer enjoyed my sport. I sswam from 4:30-6:30 a.m., played soccer from 3:00-4:00 p.m., swam again from 4:30-6:30 p.m., and then sometimes worked out again during study hall from 8:30-9:30 p.m. To the outside observer, I was the most dedicated and disciplined athlete in school. Internally, I had given up on how well I performed or competed. I trained strictly to burn calories.

My fear of food became even more pronounced mid-way through my freshman year of high school. I didn't understand beauty, but I understood that I wanted to be prettier. My family raised me to believe that I was pretty, but why didn't the boys I liked think I was stunning? Why didn't my athletic, toned body fit into size 2? In my mind, my beauty was based on being a good athlete. At Chatham Hall, I discovered for the first time that not everyone was even interested in sports, let alone impressed by someone who was a great competitor. It was culture shock – I was no longer the best, and realized that there were more things than just swimming to be the best at.

I found myself surrounded by wealthy girls. Their wardrobes and horses alone amounted to more than my family's annual income.

I discovered that my hand-me-downs, Goodwill bargains, and occasional trendy pair of jeans from Express made me the odd girl out. I craved to be beautiful too, beautiful like the rich girls who all the Woodberry Forest boys liked.

I became a social sponge: I started observing and mimicking every aspect of the high school social scene unfolding before me. The girls who got the most attention and who were the most popular wore size 0-4 in J.Crew and Lily Pulitzer, and thought of such high-end labels as mere lounge clothes. They used daddy's credit card every weekend and showered themselves with mail-ordered shopping sprees. Many times, if they didn't like what they had ordered once it arrived, they would kindly and generously pass it along to me instead of bothering to mail it back to the company. Therefore, to have stylish clothes, albeit throw-away items with the tags still on, I needed to be the same size as the skinny rich girls. At lunch, they were the girls who counted calories and used coffee cup saucers their salads. I watched the relationship of fear-respect these girls had with food and I sought that disciplinary tension too. I fervently sought out advice from classmates on the tricks to bulimia, fad diets, and appetite control. Answers were readily available.

In high school, I didn't know I was pretty. I knew I was cute, but, in my mind, I was the farthest thing from pretty. I dulled my beauty with big sporty sweatshirts and baggy shorts, and refused to wear make-up. I was an athlete, wasn't I? It was a great excuse. I feared men, only because I didn't trust the ones that found me beautiful. And beautiful, they eventually found me. I dated every cute guy I wanted; I was never dumped, never denied, and always spoiled. I ended every relationship I ever had, and I did it to preserve my ability to stay in the shadows. I convinced myself that these reputably "hot guys" didn't really want me or find me attractive, but simply couldn't find anyone else who was relatively eye-catching. I thought I was their consolation prize.

Think for a moment about how many self-loathing thoughts you allow yourself to think every day. Go ahead, stop and think; make an estimate.

Your mind controls your view of life. Have you or are you going to allow negative thoughts about yourself to dominate your thought patterns, and subsequently your life?

There was a point in my life that the extra quarter-inch of fat between my chest and my armpits consumed me. I called it my boob fat, and I hated it. Boob fat and the tiniest bit of lower tummy bulge almost destroyed me as a person. I give you my personal example just to demonstrate how absurdly selfish and neurotic the thorn in your own side might be in reality, as well. When I woke up in the morning, I would be nervous before I stepped in front of a mirror, then I would stare at myself naked, in hatred. Those were my bad days. If luck would have it that my stomach looked better in the light one morning, it would be a good day.

My view of myself in a mirror became my worldview.

I pinched myself in the places I hated, yelled at myself, and criticized my body shape. I was convinced that my life would be perfect if only those two parts of my body changed. If I looked bloated one day, I would cry in anger and frustration and allow it to ruin my day.

I know I am not alone in such a neurotic struggle.

I have spoken to and watched hundreds of women caught in a self-imposed need for some undetermined, unattainable standard of physical perfection. I have met some of the angriest gentle people in the world through my work with this struggle. Women and men who abuse themselves mentally are no different than abusers. Abuse impairs judgment and prevents growth. When you mentally abuse yourself and are overly critical of your body, you confine yourself to a prison of pain.

I often ask my clients who are too hard on themselves if they would ever dare direct some of the things they say to themselves to anyone else. They are aghast at my suggestion, for of course they wouldn't speak to anyone else with such criticism. How can we stand by and allow ourselves to speak so unkindly to our own souls?

How many of us see ourselves in a twisted manner? Do we really think that we are beautiful or do we just sometimes feel beautiful when our husbands, boyfriends, and friends tell us so?

If you think you are ugly or average, it will become a self-fulfilling prophecy. Others won't see it; just you, and you will subconsciously downplay your attributes and learn ways to hide the true, confident, fabulous *you*! If you *think* you are pretty, *you will be pretty*! Life is truly 95% mental. You are what you think. The greatest human ability is our ability to choose and to think; you have the choice and power to control your thoughts. It takes great discipline and great desire.

In a recent survey by a leading women's magazine, women were asked to rate their own attractiveness based on a 1-10 scale, with 10 being the highest. Only 3% of women believed themselves to be a 10. Most respondents feared rating themselves at the higher end of the scale. The majority of answers (a surprising 67%) reveal that American women rate themselves only between a 4 and a 7. Imagine! Beautiful, stunning women surround us, but most of them are strangers to their own beauty. In any given day at the gym, I interact with at least 100 women whom I deem above-average in beauty and uniqueness; it is distressing to think that 67 of those 100 consider themselves simply "average."

It astonishes me how, so much like myself in high school, we are afraid of our own beauty. We are afraid to feel sexy or to admit that we feel pretty one day. Author Jane Rubietta states: "How we actually look is less important than how we *think* we look." How fittingly true.

A recent study unveiled more interesting statistics. Globally, out of the millions interviewed internationally in hundreds of languages, only two percent elected to describe themselves with the adjective *beautiful*. Angelina Jolie, considered by many to be the most beautiful woman in the world, is no different from the average in the way she perceives herself. She confessed: "I struggle with low self-esteem all the time. I think everyone does. I have so much wrong with me, it's unbelievable."

So, how do we escape this seemingly pervasive plight of women? We learn, like the French, to love food. We learn to love our imperfections. We learn that the beauty of our personalities sparkles through our eyes when we smile with confidence. We learn to think beautiful thoughts.

It's time to learn to think beautiful thoughts. Make a list of ten expressive adjectives about yourself. Be specific, be thoughtful, and do not be afraid to be proud of your beauty. Share your list with someone and do not be embarrassed of your open praises of yourself. Write them in the box provided and review your list frequently.

The more you meditate on a thought, the more naturally your subconscious mind will deem it to be true. Your subconscious mind does not interpret information, but simply takes it as fact. Thanks to many years of psychological study, we know that the human brain is capable of unbelievable feats when the power of the subconscious is properly trained and activated. A woman with a *skinny mind* will take the power of the sub-conscious and run with it, for she knows that her subconscious will transform her confidence, beauty, and enjoyment of life.

BEAUTIFUL THOUGHTS
TO ACTIVATE THE CONFIDENT
SUB-CONSCIOUS

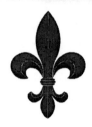

1. _____

2. _____

3. _____

4. _____

5. _____

6. _____

7. _____

8. _____

9. _____

10. _____

YOU AND OTHERS

My childhood echoes with my mother's refrain: "Garbage in, garbage out." I don't think that she realized the philosophical depth of the popular proverb beyond the moral sense. For so many years, I didn't get it, though I do now. The French get it, too.

Our French sisters simply don't let the garbage of negative self-talk into their subconscious. They embrace their unique physical blemishes, they add funk to their fashion, and make little black dresses seem personalized to express themselves. Uniqueness is praised and appreciated. They understand that perfumeries exist because each scent smells so distinctively beautiful and different on each person's skin, with each person's chemical balance. It is a *petit luxe* of both science and art. They read French *Glamour* and French *Cosmo* for fashion and nutritional trends, without turning to Hollywood for ideas. Dr. Susie Orbache, psychotherapist and professor at the London School of Economics, discovered that, after spending less than five minutes reading a fashion magazine, over eighty percent of women demonstrated lower self-esteem. Garbage in, garbage out.

In my mid-twenties, I caught myself baffled by my own beauty. I couldn't stop taking pictures of my new boyfriend and myself. Sounds egocentric, but it was sincere shock. Such shock, in fact, that I attributed the attractiveness and confidence that I saw in myself to him; he, a former model, chose me and therefore validated my own beauty. After so many years of self-deception and lies (otherwise known as mental garbage) to myself, I couldn't believe that I was the beautiful woman smiling so strikingly in the photographs. Still muddied in my thinking, I recognized that I was starting to feel sexy but I wasn't sure if it was because of him or because of me.

I was in a battle of deciphering the "garbage out." Truthfully, I was captivated by myself. My beauty not only enthralled me, but also confused me. I saw myself as a woman for the first time. I could not comprehend, though, what this attractive man saw in me. I wrote off my bewilderment, distracted myself by focusing on how lucky I was to be his "chosen one," and called it love.

Fifteen months later, I began to see things more clearly. It took me experiencing a tumultuous, toxic relationship where I considered myself unworthy in level of attractiveness to finally realize that *I* was the one that was truly beautiful inside and out. *I* drew people to me, without his help.

Retrospectively, I recognize that as a period of ambiguous self-admiration. It was my coming of age; my metamorphosis of self-discovery. Once you have a positive mindset of self-acceptance, looking at old pictures is one of the healthiest forms of positive body activism one can engage in. Months after a photo is taken, you can claim a more secure ownership of your beauty, and slowly, but surely, you begin to reclaim your ability to think fabulous, pretty, less critical thoughts.

Women *are* different from men. We have a terrible ability to subconsciously analyze and judge one another upon first glance. In doing so, we sabotage ourselves. Each judgment, each observation, each critical thought about one another only makes our own body-esteem all the more vulnerable. Moreover, many of us simply don't see the real image of ourselves when we look in the mirror. We are so jaded by media images and unrealistic standards of thinness that even our reflection is unrecognizable to our own eyes. The more we criticize others in our own quest for self-affirmation, the more we destroy our own selves.

According to business etiquette and human interaction expert Lydia Ramsey, the average human interaction involves eleven judgments of the opposite person within the first seven seconds of meeting and 93% of judgment is based on non-verbal data. Seemingly innocent, simple, unspoken observations ultimately take on a morphing nature within the psyche. The internal dialogue of comments and judgments about clothes, body type, hair, and accessories are innate in many women. Every time that this subconscious dialogue takes a critical spin, one allows and invites reverse judgment upon themselves, most of which actually comes from within.

Researchers estimate that approximately 87% of all communication is non-verbal. So then, if the majority of communication with others is non-verbal, it can be assumed that self-reflective communication is primarily non-verbal as well.

The mind is the most powerful thing on earth; its power is limitless and its influence on the psyche is immeasurable. Body confidence and a lifestyle of fitness begin with the self-talk that goes on in the mind. You believe what you think, and you have the power to control the thoughts you think. You have the power harness and train your own psychological strength, that is, only if you pay enough attention to the thoughts you allow to shape your life.

We are faced with a generation of young women who think that beauty is what they see in photo-shopped magazines and in anorexic runway models. Those thoughts develop into beliefs, and non-verbal self-comparison takes place. Comparisons inevitably end with a need for physical improvement and general discontentment with our natural bodies.

Our society has manipulated the vision and focus of our lives, and we are the ones who have allowed it. Remember, we *do* have control over what we think. We have the power to choose what our aim in life is and what it is that will make us feel fulfilled and complete. Sadly, many of us buy into the idea that a perfect body will bring us great happiness.

I spent years of my life prescribing to this hope for the physical ideal, and every year that passed, my discontentment with myself only deepened. The closer I got objectively to my idea of physical perfection, the farther away I found myself from being content. This phenomenon is extremely common among perfectionists and dieters – and, well, Americans in general.

In France I learned that if your entire life vision is physically based, then your joy will also be physically based. I discovered that physical perfection is unattainable and therefore will never bring me the joy that I sought so desperately. What we must remind ourselves is that ultimately, no matter what you believe, the physical fails and the material deteriorates.

Henry Ford knew the power of the mind and of non-verbal self-talk. He famously stated: "Whether you think you can, or whether you think you can't, you are right." Let me rephrase that for those of us fighting to embrace ourselves and to develop a lasting, genuine body-confidence: Whether you think you are beautiful, or whether you think you aren't, you are right.

Every woman I met in France knew she was beautiful. Based on my experience, this is what I have found, and I found it incredibly beautiful and inspiring. It was like living confidently in their own skin was enmeshed with their nature. They were born with it; or rather, their society is structured so that they grow in confident individuality and beauty. Even the pimply, awkward teenagers that I taught in Périgueux had body confidence that is hard to come by in the States. Be honest with yourself: know that life is but a vapor. Not embracing it because you cannot embrace your body is tragic. In fact, hating your own skin is a self-destructive tragedy that kills the soul and true spirit of a being.

Body confidence is a *choice*. It is an individual's decision to embrace and accept his or her physical stature, shape, and unique features. Once you commit yourself to a lifestyle of self-acceptance, you are on your way to true beauty."

I believe that body confidence begins with corrective posture changes. Enter a room proudly and be accepting of your body how it is. Try it; you will be amazed at the way your thought patterns about yourself will change. It's remarkable, the power of unspoken communication. The impact of body language is evident not only on others, but also on you personally. Try the following experiment and you may even surprise yourself.

Here's the challenge: spend three days focusing entirely on your posture. Feel each individual vertebra elongate and breathe in deeply through your nose and exhale slowly through your mouth. When you inhale, allow the air to fill your lungs, and as you exhale out tighten your abs and core. Conscientious breathing will help you become more aware of your body and posture; the more aware you are of yourself, the more you will begin to appreciate yourself. Look at people directly in the eyes and avoid darting your gaze away from anyone. Proudly keep your shoulders back, chest out, and chin up.

It will be difficult for you to not feel confident as you continue the experiment. People may ask you if you have lost weight. Others will notice that you seem self-assured and may even note that you seem subtly happier. It is this astute happiness that makes French women so undeniably sexy and mysterious. They walk with pride and confidence because they have mastered ownership of their posture and body.

On the fourth day, allow yourself to slouch. Do it for an hour, either while you are driving, or watching TV. Walk around a bit; be as comfortable and slouchy as possible. Afterwards, try to evaluate how you feel. Most of my clients who have done this experiment note that they feel achy and lethargic when they slouch. Some comment that they feel more down on themselves when they slouch and even noticed how their tummy pouched out more on day four. Just seeing the difference in body posture and the effect it had on their overall body confidence made them more prone to unhealthy food and fitness choices.

Remember, the way you present yourself to others is your choice. Keep in mind that also affects how you present yourself to yourself. *Own* your beauty and your health. Your health is your choice; your body does not lie. Your physical well-being is a direct reflection of the lifestyle choices you have made, as well as a manifestation of who you are deep down.

How many days have you woken up and found your mind thinking discontented thoughts about your body? How many years of your life have you wasted hating your body and wishing it was more like someone else's? How many times can you recall saying "I just wish [*insert such and such physical attribute*] was thinner, fuller, longer, sleeker, firmer, or shaped differently?" For each moment you allow your mind to drift to those places of self-betrayal and discontentment, you affect your body-confidence. I am noticeably distracted and self-conscious when my thoughts are flooded with *"I wishes"* and *"if only's"* about my body. It saddens me to think how many hours and days of my life I have wasted by simply being too lazy or too weak to control my own thought patterns.

Many of us in America are so driven that we live our lives focused on what we don't have and on what we need to achieve. It is said that if you look at what you do not have in life, you don't have anything. If you look at what you do have in life, you have everything. The same maybe said of health and beauty. If we spend our days focused on what we don't have physically and on how to perfect our external beauty, then we will never be authentically beautiful. Those women who believe fundamentally in their beauty have a loveliness and a body confidence that is not for purchase, that is not photo-shoppable, and that can never be taken away.

Women who build their body confidence upon positivity and self-acceptance are able to free themselves to live life as it is meant to be lived: passionately and fully. Marie Jose Maripec, an elite French athlete, summarizes this secret to French fitness in four simple words: *"vivre à votre rythme,"* which translates to "live life at your rhythm."

The key to living life at your own rhythm is to control the observations and judging thoughts you have about others. Look instead for ways to verbally affirm and compliment others. In building up others, you will begin also to allow more positive thoughts to drift toward yourself. Find five things each day to compliment yourself and others on and be distinct enough in your body language that your body confirms the statements.

Society thrives on categorizing individuals into larger groups in order to make sense of the multitude of personalities and body types, and to establish social status. Allowing yourself to be involved in labeling, which is practically an inevitable experience that we all encounter in life, can be one of the most self-destructive choices you can make. When you subscribe to being labeled, whether you are described as preppy, emo, sporty, trendy, or whatever category, you limit yourself and you lose sight of yourself. Boxing yourself up by identifying with a certain type of crowd inevitably changes your focus to living for others. You try to fit in and try to blend in. It is as if you are tying up your hands and preventing yourself to be free in your individualism. It is daunting to stand alone and be contently unique, but it is a necessary step in learning to understand *you*.

It may be helpful to dissect some specific examples of people who limit themselves. Who are the people in your life that you are most desperately trying to impress? Why does their opinion matter so much to you that you will rearrange your actions and appearance around what they expect? Are there people in your life that make you feel insecure? Who are those people and why do they hold a power of criticism and judgment over you? Finally, consider the people in your life that make you feel empowered and confident in simply being *you*. What is the difference between these people and the people you are desperate to impress?

If your answers reveal conflicts and misperceptions in your life, you are not alone. Consider whether it would be more freeing to not fit than to strive to belong.

Rosie, one of my clients from Wisconsin, struggles like many of us do. She is a fair-skinned, fit surgical assistant who used to be a personal trainer. Married to a plastic surgeon, Rosie bears the self-imposed cross of looking perfect. One day, mid-workout and winded, Rosie muttered a simple, yet profound statement that represents the crux of this chapter. As she rolled up her black spandex Capris, she unveiled the thorn in her side: scarred marks on the back of her toned thighs from a pregnancy-related emergency. She gasped in her sweet Kentucky way: "I just can't walk around like this when people know that I am married to a plastic surgeon. I know it doesn't matter, but I buy into their judgment and I impose it upon myself. My poor husband just doesn't understand." She refuses to wear a swimsuit and fears putting on shorts.

Rosie's statement rocked me and it made me think about how I label myself and how I label others. We tend to compartmentalize ourselves in order to find a social grouping into which we "fit." It makes us feel accepted. It makes us feel normal, or so we think. I am the fit, blonde and tan personal trainer. Rosie is the plastic surgeon's wife. Libby is the All-American sorority girl who dates only fraternity guys. Gabby is an American Sign Language interpreter who sometimes refuses to speak in order to fit more fully into the deaf community. Holly is the granola girl that preaches more about eating organic and going green than she practices.

We all just want to fit somewhere. We all just want to be accepted. Why don't we start with just accepting ourselves first? We don't need to rely on other's labels of us to empower our place in society or our true identity. As Danish philosopher Soren Kierkegaard profoundly stated, "If you label me, you negate me."

Let's investigate further into what labeling really does and let's stop allowing ourselves to be labeled:

As a personal trainer, I used to feel a certain unspoken pressure when in social situations. On the beach, I was embarrassed if my abs were not as chiseled as Jillian Michaels'. At a restaurant, I could never eat without someone commenting on the healthy choice that I had made. An introduction of myself as a personal trainer was sure to result in some sort of touching of my body or comment on how strong I must be. I needed to fit the profile. I wanted to fit the profile, even though I understood and tried to cling to the value of my unique individuality.

Refuse to be labeled; doing so begins with not labeling yourself first. Categorizing yourself as independent and unique is among the most freeing things you can do for yourself. Live and be you. Stop worrying about others' perceptions of you and what crowd you most identify with; all that labeling does for you is to restrict the full vibrancy of your identity. Labeling not only limits you for reaching your full potential in confidence and self-awareness, but it prevents you from discovering the intricacies that make you *you*.

We should all strive to be consistent in our beings. Our outward appearance reflects what occupies our minds on the inside.

Water your mind with seeds of strength. Identify the areas of your thought-life that ultimately end up bringing you down; weed out those weaknesses one by one as you focus on your personal growth. Remember, in life you are growing, regressing, or stagnating.

Be the type of person people admire – be a lifelong self-learner. Nothing is more humbling, more prosperous, nor more satisfying. Be generous. Whether you believe in karma or The Golden Rule, you will always reap what you sow. So sow generously, and you will reap generously. Sow sparingly, and you will harvest nothing. Usually we use this analogy in relationships with others, but in order to arrive at a loving acceptance of yourself, you must sow generously in the direction of your own development.

Everything discussed in this book will not happen overnight. Changes will not happen by chance, nor will they happen without discipline of thought and dedication to persistence in implementing positive mind patterns. Be generous to yourself and invest in taking time to really hone your perspective on life and on yourself. If you do not take this time for yourself, you will never truly change. There are endless ways to sow your own seeds of growth: journaling, reading, yoga, meditation, stretching, writing, painting, sewing, and exercising to clear your mind, just to name a few.

You *must* slow down and you must clear your mind and allow it to reflect. The creativity and peacefulness you allow yourself will prepare your mind to be pliable and cleansed. These moments to yourself are intimate and potentially the most self-awakening moments you will ever experience. In taking time for yourself, you will finally have the ability to listen to and actually *hear* your inner voice. You will learn what you really desire and, in such quietness, what really makes your heart come alive.

Quiet time, whatever your preferred method, can prove to be the pivotal point in the development of your own self-empowerment. As you start to understand yourself, you will start to appreciate yourself. This step of self-appreciation will transform your ability to really start loving yourself. Once you start loving yourself, you have hit a goldmine and you will discover the hidden gems inside of you that you never knew existed.

YOU AND THE MIRROR.
Skinny, Sexy *à la carte*
L'herbe est toujours plus verte chez le voisin.
[The grass is always greener on the other side.]

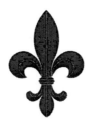

i. Skinny, Sexy SUMMARY:

The mirror can betray and distort both our self perception and self-value. We often don't see ourselves for how we actually look, so be careful in believing the mirror and in giving it any power in your life.

Our society has manipulated the vision and focus of our lives, and we are the ones who have allowed it. Remember, we are beautiful *because* of our distinct uniqueness, and we do have control over what we think.

ii. Skinny, Sexy REFLECTIONS:

Do you avoid mirrors? How do "bad" photos make you feel? *Does your mirror, or perhaps the scale, control your worldview?* Are you ready to start saying kinder words to yourself about the image you see in the mirror? *Do you choose your thoughts daily?* Body confidence is a *choice* - do you choose it? *Are you generous to yourself or only generous to others?* What do you love to do? What hobbies make you come alive?

iii. Skinny, Sexy PRACTICAL APPLICATION:

Be French - tell yourself that you're sexy every time you look in a mirror, no matter how "sexy" you actually do or don't feel.

Posture practice! Watch your feet while you stand, walk and sit. Try to keep everything in a neutral alignment; doing so will permit your body weight to stay in an optimal muscular equilibrium. French women are known for great, sexy posture. Sloppy, slouchy posture just isn't sexy. Stand up straight and you will look like you have lost five pounds instantly. Try to be aware of your breathing; this will increase your self-awareness. The more aware you are of yourself, the more you will begin to appreciate yourself and to stop comparing yourself to others.

iv. Skinny, Sexy EATING:

The food you put into your body mirrors how you will feel in your body. Eat whole, natural, unprocessed foods and you will start feeling sexier from the inside out.

v. Skinny, Sexy YOU:

Put positive Post-its on the mirror around your house and in your car until you start accepting the perfectly imperfection image you see.

Be a life-long self learner.

Shower others in authentic compliments and refuse to allow your mind to criticize others for this will only come back to you.

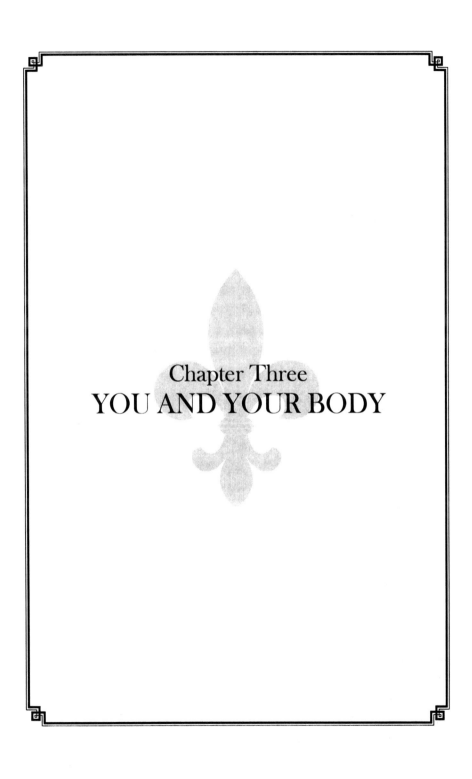

Chapter Three
YOU AND YOUR BODY

Chapter Three
YOU AND YOUR BODY

One of the most defining and important relationships in your life is between you and your body. Many people are not aware of this relationship, though it exists in everyone. There are a variety of factors that go into creating an understanding of this relationship: societal pressures, interpersonal relationships, and physical and psychological implications. Everyone's mind-body awareness begins at some point in their childhood and evolves from there, depending on the factors of his/her environment. Essentially, your relationship with your body is birthed at the moment you realize that your body is different from others'. It is the point at which you start to decide whether or not you like the skin you are in. You register how it feels to be you, and you start to notice and listen to what others around you say and imply about you and your body. For many of us, we develop a negative relationship with the image of our body at some point.

When did your feelings about your body become negative? Identify that pivotal moment in your life. Was it during your childhood, or perhaps your adulthood? I remember the birth of my negative body relationship: I had two moments. The first was when I was eight. I was playing with my brother's two friends on the playground before swim practice. I was hanging upside down on the monkey bars and suddenly my shirt went over my head, exposing my flat chest. The two little boys I was with laughed at me and made jokes about me still being a little girl; they said I would never have boobs and that I would never be one of the girls that the boys liked. I remember laughing them off and then spending that entire night alone in my room, staring at my body in the mirror. For years, I thought I would never become a woman.

The comments we hear when we are young have a profound impact on us that most don't recognize.

My second revelation came in high school, when I was a sophomore. One of my best friends, who incidentally was much thinner than I was, started throwing up every meal she ate. I was confused for a few weeks about why she was doing what she was doing. Then one day I tried to borrow her clothes for a dance we had with a local boys' school and I was disgusted with myself to find out that I didn't fit into the size 2 shirt of hers I wanted to wear. She suggested that I become bulimic, told me it was super easy, and promised me that it would give me the perfect body. She coached me for a few weeks, gave me some of her clothes, and introduced me to diet pills.

Author Mary Pipher describes this "ah-ha" moment of awful discovery as pivotal in the mental development of youth and their relationships with not only their bodies, but with their entire identity. In her book, *Reviving Ophelia: Saving the Selves of Adolescent Girls* she describes the dissatisfaction that a young girl experiences during puberty in modern, media-saturated America:

> Just at the point that their bodies are becoming rounder, girls are told that thin is beautiful, even imperative. Girls hate the required gym classes in which other girls talk about their fat thighs and stomachs. One girl told me of showering next to an eighty-five-pound dancer who was on a radical diet. For the first time in her life she looked at her body and was displeased.

In contemplating Pipher's words, what feelings come to mind when you remember your adolescent years? How did your body image develop during those years? Remember, every part of our being is in continual development and evolution – try to identify the journey of you and your body.

Another imperative question to ask is what voices in your life have impacted the way you view yourself and your body? For me, the voices of my cool bulimic friend and two nine-year-old boys ring in my ears. The voices tell me over and over again that my body will never measure up to perfection and that I will never be beautiful enough. Perhaps you have voices of family members suggesting that you diet, or a coach who called you fat in front of your peers. Whatever your voices, we all have them. It is up to you to recognize and silence those voices so that your own voice can take off and be free.

Nicole Johnson, author of *A Fresh Brewed Life* wrote about the impact of such voices. She says, "These voices keep our souls chained in the basement. They make us fearful to try anything new, anxious about what others think of us, and they keep us on the treadmill of performance."

Johnson is so right. These voices keep us on "the treadmill of performance," or the treadmill of perfection. This treadmill is a never ending effort to please others that ultimately gets you nowhere. To silence the voices and get off the treadmill, you have to value who you are as a person. The voices of others should not define your identity and relationship with your body. Your voice is the defining one, so stop letting other's opinions bully you around; start giving yourself a voice again.

Women desire beauty because we listen to the messages of the world that say it will bring us power and control. This is a myth and a materialistic misconception that makes us resign and give our hearts away. We are living in a society that is fat-phobic and prejudiced towards those who are overweight. Sadly, the more obsessed we become with avoiding these qualities, the higher our eating disorder and obesity rates rise. This battle for our bodies is about more than food, exercise, and dieting; this is about a state of mind and being. Freedom from the hamster wheel that our nation's health is stuck on is found in the redefinition of our body image. Body-critiquing will stop as soon as you realize whether or not you are afraid of being fat and unhealthy or whether you are simply afraid of society's harsh judgment.

The key to mastering a *skinny, sexy mind* is found not in the transformation of the body, but in the transformation of the mind. Another way to evolve in the transformation of your mind is to re-evaluate how you think your body should look. Your goal should never to be thin, but to be healthy. Part of the secret of a *skinny, sexy mind* is found in understanding that "skinny" is a word relative to each individual body.

Your external features, body type, style, and physical characteristics reveal nothing of the true you. Your outward appearance and your body tell the world nothing of your passions, dreams, hobbies, hopes, or personality. That is why beauty on the outside is only as beautiful and powerful as you are on the inside.

Take time to think about how you feel from the inside out. Now. Slowly. Put the book down for a minute, an hour, or a day and think. Now that you have identified the voices of your past that you have allowed to dominate your self-image, it is time to erase those voices and re-establish your external image from an internal standpoint. So, how do you feel in the skin you are in? What does it feel like to be you and why is that wonderfully unique? Remember, the way you feel in your skin will be the foundation of your body image; your body is your vessel of transportation in the world, not your identity. Examples of what it might feel like to be in your skin could be some of the following adjectives: alive, tingly, firm, content, comfortable, at ease, confident, tall, relaxed, vibrant, and healthy.

In the previous chapter, we learned about the power the mirror has over our self-image. Similarly, when you look in a mirror, look at your whole body. Do not break your body apart. Do not allow your eyes to wander to only one area of your body, for this is not how the world sees you. See yourself as a whole; see your entire body. In doing so, you will begin to identify yourself as whole.

Try this out for yourself. Stand fully naked in a mirror for five minutes. At first, stare at the part(s) of your body that you are apt to criticize, and then stare at yourself as a whole. Squint your eyes and allow your vision to become fuzzy to be able to see the whole. Now, as you look at yourself as a whole reflection, tell yourself how much you *like* that part of you that you had picked out to critique. Yes, you find that part of you *beautiful*. And, no, it does not look like the same part that you may see on a supermodel but remember, you (and three billion other women) weren't made to look like that. You look how you look for a reason; the sooner you embrace your perceived body flaws, the sooner you will have a *skinny, sexy mind*.

I urge you: embrace your uniqueness and your physical "flaws." I use quotations in saying flaws, because a physical flaw doesn't really exist. They are self-created limitations in which we prevent ourselves from being comfortable in the skin we are in.

Changing your thought life with regard to your body image is a difficult task, but with the right amount of persistence, it can and must be done. You must be patient with yourself and keep in mind that your subconscious has been repeating the same negative message to your body for years. You have to overpower the negative with a positive, and it starts with simple, repeated affirmation.

Accept yourself for how you are *now*. Repeat positive statements to yourself, even if it feels like you are lying to yourself, until the lie becomes a truth. Tell yourself, "I love my _____ (thighs, hair, bottom, eyes, knees, hips, arms, breasts, shoulders, teeth, etc.).” Substitute the word “beautiful” in lieu of whatever adjective you normally use before describing these parts of your body. Repeat the phrase ten times a day, for three weeks. You will be amazed at the way your mind changes, and the way your eyes see yourself progresses.

You will prevail because body image is a mind game, and you can choose to win. How you play determines how you win your own personal battles. It all starts with a choice. You are who you *allow* yourself to be.

A genuine compliment and an affirming word can change a person’s day, and potentially his or her entire life. It can save someone’s life because it empowers one’s inner identity, which then makes his or her body image free and alive. Never underestimate the power of a kind word.

I have had the pleasure of encountering someone who lives and breathes that motto; a co-worker of mine named Heidi affirms people on a daily basis. She is an inspiration of the power of kindness and selflessness. It is neither overt, nor fake when Heidi tells you that you look beautiful that day. She finds something striking and positive in everyone that passes her desk. I have observed and watched the unveiling of strangers’ faces upon an interaction with Heidi; people transform in front of her. She finds something unique and exquisitely beautiful in every person that passes, and, she *expresses* her admiration to them.

Now, many of us see beautiful things in one another, but honestly, how often do we verbally tell them what beauty we see? People need to hear it, everyone in a different, very personal way. Some call these kinds of encouraging people builder-uppers; I call them box-breakers. Heidi not only breaks people out of their boxes, and makes them feel loved and comfortable, but she also breaks free of the box of labels that so many of us put ourselves into.

I experimented one full week trying to emulate Heidi. Not only was I in a better mood, but everyone around me was, too. Try it out for yourself; you will be amazed at what it does for others, and what it does to your body relationship, as well. It was astounding that in complimenting other people, and really seeking out true beauty in every person I interacted with, that I too felt more beautiful. I felt sexy on my most bloated day of the week. I was joyful when my caffeine buzz wore off and energy depleted. It was probably the most enjoyable, yet busiest work weeks I have ever had. Love attracts love, and as beauty is revealed, the soul is freed into buoyant exuberance. Within a day, my entire staff of fifty was showering one another and one another's clients in compliments. The most baffling part of it all: none of it was forced or seemed fake.

When you come from a place of love, love spreads. The love inside you will grow and flourish in parallel with the growth and development of your self-image. The more in tune you are with yourself, the beauty of your body as it is today, and the wonderful attributes that make you *you*, the more your openness and confidence will inspire and empower others. Your beauty is a state of mind, not a state of body. Once you accept that as fact, you will feel as I felt in France: free, alive, and confident in your skin.

Authenticity stands for itself. An authentic compliment and genuine caring for others can never be criticized or negated. Focusing on others in such a humble, uplifting way will bring you to a pasture of enlightenment. Your attitude in life will shift. When you pour love into others and build them up in your care, you eliminate any seeds of jealousy and competition that may have had the potential to exist. When you learn to free yourself from the internal need to impress or compete with others, then you will begin to learn the true art of living. Protest the messages and voices in your life that make you think negatively about your body. Become a critic of attitudes, media publications, and societal trends. Keep your mind focused on the joy of being fully you, free from the judgment and unattainable standards of society. Overwrite every negative thought concerning your body with a positive one. You will be transformed before your own eyes and others will notice the change in your confidence. Once you arrive at the "love" stage in your relationship with your body, you will exude beauty in ways you never have before.

The art of living involves so much joy, so much self-acceptance, and so much freedom that your disordered relationship with food and with your body will begin to slowly dissipate once you pursue living at your own rhythm.

IN MY SKIN, I FEEL:

1. _____

2. _____

3. _____

4. _____

5. _____

AMERICAN WOMEN: BODY IMAGE STATISTICS

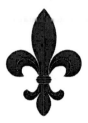

• Models weigh 23% less than the average woman. Twenty years ago, they weighed 8% less.

• The average American woman is 5'4" and weighs 140 pounds. The average American model is 5'11" and weighs 117 pounds.

• Americans spend more than 40 billion dollars a year on dieting and diet-related products – that's roughly equivalent to the amount the U.S. Federal Government spends on education each year!

• Almost half of all female smokers smoke because they see it as the best way to control their weight. Of these women, 25% will die of a disease caused by smoking.

• In 2007, there were about 11.7 million cosmetic procedures performed in the U.S. Ninety one percent of these procedures were performed on women.

• A study found that 53% of thirteen-year-old American girls are unhappy with their bodies. This number grows to 78% by the time girls reach seventeen.

• "Attractiveness Messages" bombard our youth. A study of 4,294 network television commercials revealed that one out of every 3.8 commercials send one of these messages. The average adolescent sees over 5,260 "attractiveness messages" per year.

• A survey of formerly fat people revealed they would rather be blind or lose a limb than be fat again. A similar survey revealed that women feared being fat more than dying.

• One in four college-aged women has an eating disorder. In addition, 50% of college-aged women have a disordered body image. The statistics for underweight males with negative body images parallels that of overweight women with disordered eating. Disordered eating is not gender-specific.

• Marilyn Monroe wore a size 14; most American women strive to be a size 4. Fifty percent of American women admit to being on a diet at present.

• Store mannequins in stores would be too thin to menstruate if they were alive.

• A teen magazine surveyed readers to find out why they exercised: 74% exercised "to become more attractive" and 51% stated that they also exercised to lose weight and burn calories.

YOU AND YOUR BODY.

Skinny, Sexy *à la carte*

Il faut de tout pour faire un monde.
[It takes all sorts to make a world.]

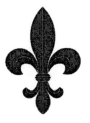

i. Skinny, Sexy SUMMARY:

The relationship between you and your body can determine everything about the way you live your life.

ii. *Skinny, Sexy REFLECTIONS:*

Are you *biens dans votre peau? Do you like the skin you are in? What phrases and thoughts inhibit you from* being able to accept your body? *Can you remember the moment that you realized that your body wasn't "perfect" according to societal standards?* What voices in your life have affected the way you view yourself and your body?

iii. *Skinny, Sexy PRACTICAL APPLICATION:*

Write all memories of "negative voices" down, make a list and at the bottom write: "these do not define or affect me. I am perfect the way I am today." Make a commitment to verbally compliment others on a more frequent basis. Be a builder-upper and see how it starts to make you feel sexier.

iv. *Skinny, Sexy EATING:*

Resist the temptation to indulge in emotional eating. Food should never be used as a punishment or a reward; as is food is a basic simple pleasure of life. Engaging in emotional eating will lead to binging and purging and an imbalanced relationship and control of food.

v. *Skinny, Sexy YOU*

Reflect upon your *rhythm de vivre* and on how you would like to continue to live. Only you have the power to change the things about your life that you want to change. Don't wait or be dissatisfied with your quality of living if you aren't willing to start making your life and your body your own.

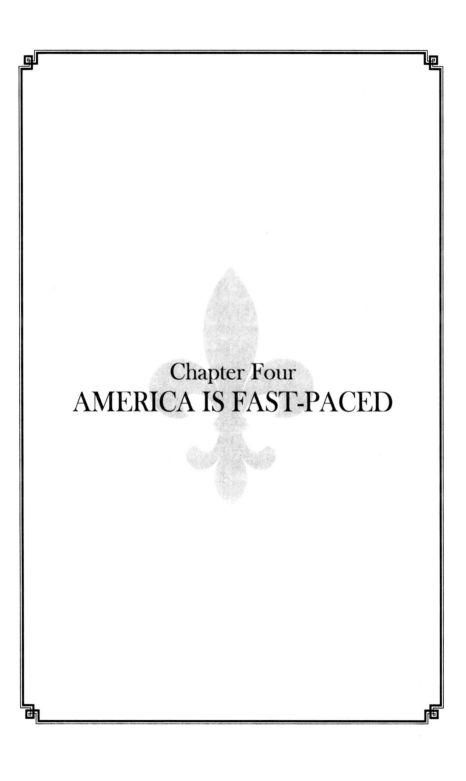

Chapter Four
AMERICA IS FAST-PACED

Chapter Four
AMERICA IS FAST-PACED

In America, we just don't have time. America prides itself on multi-tasking, mass-producing, and well-rounded success. We strive for perfection and we place too high of demands upon ourselves.

There are many contributing factors to this reality, but from the perspective of the health club industry and my experience as a personal trainer, I can conclude that we are suffering as a culture due to our lifestyle. Our American lives of fast food and our non-stop pace of life are making us a "fast nation" on the fast track to decline. Life in America is life on-the-go. We condition ourselves to be workaholics and we brag about how many weekly hours we spend in the office. We work 60 hour weeks, spend ten hours at the gym, volunteer for our kids' schools, take care of the house and family, and squeeze in time for a coffee at Starbucks with a friend. We overextend and exhaust ourselves.

It's no wonder that when we allow our bodies to rest, they panic. Often, we take the signs of exhaustion to be signs of hunger. Moreover, we simply don't know how to just *be.*

Believe it or not, there *is* such a thing as successfully wasting time. It is a fine art in France. It is *joie de vivre* and is a concept we will explore together in a later chapter. This joy of life comes from the accumulation of lots of *petits plaisirs*. But how do you discover your little pleasures in life if you don't ever take the time to stop and smell the roses? The answer: you don't.

In Périgueux, France, where I lived and worked post-graduation from college, I learned the decadent pleasure of spending an entire morning or afternoon at a café doing nothing. It takes patience and the ability to just *be* to fully savor the *petits plaisirs* that make life so very wonderful and sensual.

We have to learn to spoil ourselves by means other than food. We have to listen to our bodies, to be attuned to their every need, and to learn to allow them to be in balance.

If balance is something we want to achieve, we will never experience it without learning to do nothing. As far as instant gratification goes, it is definitely not a French concept. In fact, it doesn't even translate. It is in fact in denying ourselves something so that we are able to more fully appreciate it later. This is patience. Patience brings pleasure, pleasure brings satisfaction, and satisfaction brings *joie de vivre*.

Everything is connected when we allow ourselves to be in balance.

Time is the most valuable currency we have. How do you spend your time? How many hours weekly is spent between work, family, friends, pleasure, and doing nothing? Take ten minutes and break it down.

	MON	TUE	WED	THU	FRI	SAT	SUN	TOTAL
Work:								
Family:								
Errands:								
Friends:								
Pleasure:								
Exercise:								
Sleep:								

Remember, there are only 168 hours in a week. Based on your graph results above, what is it that you prioritize the most week to week? Are you surprised with your results?

Sleep is typically one of the first things we skimp on and it is one of the most essential to our health. Sleeping at least seven hours at night not only allows your body to rest and recover, but it recharges your emotions and mental well-being to be energized and present for family, friends, and work the next day. If you are foregoing sleep because you are too busy, then you are only fooling yourself. Sacrificing sleep can be one of the most damaging things we can do to ourselves. Studies have shown that the body's hormone regulation during sleep is one of the most important processes for weight management. Sleep impacts the body's regulation and balance of the hunger and the satiety hormones of leptin and grehlin; when these two hormones are out of whack, the body suffers tremendously, the thyroid is offset, and the body will naturally gain or hold on to fat in order to protect itself.

Based on your current schedule, what do you wish you could prioritize that you aren't right now? How balanced is your life and are you happy with where the majority of your hours are being spent? Time is something we can never get back. We need to live without regrets and be able to look back at the time we spent over our lives and be satisfied that we lived as we wanted to.

You can live in balance, too. It's your choice, and simply a matter of how you prioritize and break down your day. If you follow your heart and whatever makes you feel alive, chances are that you will find your own natural balance.

This is where we can emulate the French. Even though France has been notably Americanized over the past decade and city life is equally as go-go-go as in America, we can learn from the cultural base that provincial France still thrives on. The French work week caps out at 35 hours, very few companies permit overtime, and all companies grant five weeks of paid vacation to full-time employees.

The country is perpetually on *grève*, or strike, which sometimes affects the fluidity and functionality of an entire town, thereby granting the French worker even more time off.

Part of the power of the French is their mastery of contradictions. Wellness is a gray area of balance and is something that doesn't exist very naturally in American society. This unconventional paradox plays a significant role in every aspect of French culture and lifestyle and can be beautifully understood through author Debra Ollivier's explanation of *jolie-laide* beauty in her recent book *What French Women Know*:

> If French women have a certain allure, it's because they grow up in a world where cookie-cutter beauty is not exalted – a world where it's generally okay not to give a damn about being anyone other than yourself, and where nuances, gray zones, and contradictions can coexist. Contradictions like beautiful and ugly. Like *jolie* and *laide*. That they live in a culture with such a flamboyantly generous concept – that they generally reject notions of packaged beauty and packaged lives – gives them enough feminine guile and freedom to assert themselves as sensual beings whether they're classically pretty, *jolie laide*, or just Plain Jane. And that, in a word, is truly sexy.

American actress Maggie Gyllenhaal, was originally rejected by Hollywood for not being "beautiful enough. " She then famously told producers that they "must have a boring idea of what beautiful and sexy is," and her continued success in both foreign and American films demonstrates the power of this French contradiction of beauty. In France, sexy is vibrant, different, *jolie laide,* and most definitely never boring.

The French work to live, rather than live to work. I can attest to the validity of such a statement from my experience teaching in Périgueux, France. My responsibility as an *Assistant d'anglais* for the Bordeaux School Board was to engage French children into full-immersion language teaching and to be a cultural ambassador for the United States. I worked at six different schools within the town of Périgueux, teaching CM1, CM2, CE1, 5ème and 6ème, the equivalent of 2nd – 7th grades in the American educational system.

I was considered a full-time employee even though I only worked an average of 17 hours a week. My supervisor was kind enough to understand that I had neither an international drivers license nor a car, so he allowed for two to three hours of daily "commuting" for me as it required 40 minutes to walk from school to school and I was expected to split my time between an average of three to four schools a day.

My arrival at each school was like a breath of fresh air for the teachers whose classes I had come to take over for an hour. More often than not, the lead teacher would embrace me with a *bise,* and would promptly scurry out to the teacher's lounge to have coffee and a croissant, clearly thankful for a shortened work day. A few times, during an afternoon class, the teacher would run off to a late lunch with co-workers and instruct me to simply take the children out to play outside for the rest of the day. Upon the teachers' return, the children were released back to their parents, and I was invited to tea or to share a bottle of wine at the closest café to the school.

Towards the holidays, when exams and progress evaluations were due for the students, I would often arrive to teach and would be instructed that I was not needed that day. I was given a *jour ferié,* or free day, approximately twenty percent of my teaching days. Never once was my pay docked, and my supervisors would always advise me to take advantage of the *ponts* built into the bank holiday calendar. They encouraged me to travel Europe, to discover every corner of the French hexagon, and to even take an extra day off if necessary. "You only live once," they would say, "work will always be here."

To my delight, not only was I classified as a full-time employee, but I was also covered by French social services. I had my own green Carte Vitale (French health insurance card) and qualified for government assistance for housing. The French government generously requested that I pay only 15% of my rent, which totaled monthly to about 74€. The government then paid my landlady the remaining 419 € she charged for the fully-furnished studio apartment I rented. It was clear to me that attempting to work more in order to afford my entire rent was not only unnecessary, but a frivolous idea. It was as if France would laugh at me if I made any effort to break free of the mold into which I was comfortably placed.

My life in France could be outlined according to the following table. Please note that I spent zero time with family simply because they were in the United States:

	MON	TUE	WED	THU	FRI	SAT	SUN	TOTAL
Work:	4	2	4	4	3	0	0	17
Family:	0	0	0	0	0	0	0	0
Errands:	1	1	1	1	1	1	1	7
Friends:	5	6	5	5	5	10	10	46
Pleasure:	4	5	4	4	5	3	3	28
Exercise:	2	2	2	2	2	2	2	14
Sleep:	8	8	8	8	8	8	8	56

Clearly, such leisure and time with family and friends is unrealistic in American society. I am sharing it with you to help you understand the fundamental difference between working to live and living to work. That is not to say that that in America we cannot love where we work and what we do, thereby classifying work as pleasure.

I currently love my profession as a personal trainer, lifestyle fitness coach and fitness entrepreneur and I do consider working with my clients and my employees as pleasurable. However, I simply do not have the free time I did in France. I work six days a week, typically for ten hours a day, and I spend any free time I do have working out or writing.

Though it would be an impossibility to mimic the leisure I experienced in France, it *is* possible for me to incorporating certain nuggets of free living into my go-go-go American schedule. Many of us, without realizing it, become trampled by the daily grind. We don't intend to lose control of our priorities, but we sometimes forget who we are and lose our ability to self-direct. It is essential that you know yourself. By knowing yourself well, you will never get lost again. You will learn how to minimize things that are negatively dominating your life, and will have the power to spend more time doing the things you really love. If you never know what you really love to do, you will never find the way to your natural state of balance and joy.

Think about your dream life. How would your dream days realistically play out? As adults, we sometimes forget that we can live the life we dream. As children we know that the world is our oyster, but somewhere in the business of life, we forget that our dreams can be made reality if we want them to be, and believe them to be. Henry David Thoreau conveys this timeless concept eloquently and simply: "Live the life you've dreamed. Most men lead lives of quiet desperation and go to the grave with the song still in them." Thoreau knows very well the difference between living and life. Let the song out of you, live your *joie* and follow the life you've dreamed of, and I assure you that you will love the skin you are in.

With Thoreau in mind, think seriously about how you dream to fill in this chart of priorities. Include work hours, and if you are in a field you are not passionate about, also think about a career switch and what that switch would be. Make this graph a realistic representation of what you can change your life to be. Take time filling it out, and think about the small ways in which you can start restructuring your actual daily schedule to reflect what is going to make you into the balanced being you are about to become. Most importantly, do not forget the child inside you and keep Thoreau's words close to your heart and mind.

	MON	TUE	WED	THU	FRI	SAT	SUN	TOTAL
Work:								
Family:								
Errands:								
Friends:								
Pleasure:								
Exercise:								
Sleep:								

My daily life in France was so different from anything I had ever experienced that I realized that living life in such a way is a gift. Give this gift to yourself, for you are the only one who can. I was blessed that my life in France was structured in such a way that the gift arrived without my knowing it, providing more *joie* and happiness than I ever had known possible. It is no wonder that the friendships I forged and the adventures I experienced glimmer with fondness in my memory and inspire me to live the rest of my life accordingly. After France, I was able to live my life in the States as a gift, not a to-do list.

That is my challenge to you: let go of your to-do list and just live. Not only will this change your understanding of your relationship with others, but it will transform your understanding of yourself.

I believe that many Americans, and certainly some French, live their lives in such a hurried panic to get to the "next step" that they never slow down to taste what life really has to offer.

Soren Kierkegaard philosophized on this very subject of life pace and pleasure in saying that "most men pursue pleasure with such breathless haste that they hurry past it." Possibly the most fitting an ubiquitous example of this is the role of fast food in our lives. Manufactured and marketed to appeal to our youth – the average American child sees 7,600 fast food advertisements per year – the fast food chains prey on the non-stop lifestyle of Americans, and the French as well. Fast food is the easy answer for the stressed-out, time-constrained working parent. Fast food lures people into its trap of convenience and economy before taking its tragic effect.

The inconvenient truth is that healthy food not only takes more time to prepare and shop for, but it is significantly more expensive. I tell my clients to shop the perimeter of the grocery store, to buy organic, and to avoid anything with more than five ingredients listed. Most are able to follow these simple instructions and benefit tremendously from the dietary change. Unfortunately, their grocery bill is much higher. The backwards state of our industrialized food industry is that two-liter bottles of sugary soda, bags of greasy chips, and other packaged snacks are under two dollars whereas a fresh head of broccoli can cost over three dollars. It is no wonder that the unhealthy food wins out in many American's shopping carts.

Nor is it any wonder that so many Americans are addicted to foods that are high in saturated fat, low in quality carbohydrates, and high in sodium. The American food industry has perverted much of our understanding of what "good" food is and isn't. We spend millions of dollars annually on calorie-controlled frozen diet meals that are overloaded with sodium as a preservative, and we wonder why we keep getting fatter, and encountering higher blood pressure and more heart attacks. The amount of sodium intake in the typical American diet is more than double what the FDA recommends. The unhealthy effects of high sodium are causing the FDA to consider regulating sodium.

Fast food, whether it is from the frozen food section, a drive-through window, or a chain restaurant is not only nutrient-void, but has gone from being an occasional treat to a staple in many Americans' diets.

Convenience stores and gas stations are no different. I can still remember the wonder, as a child, of stepping into a 7-Eleven with my father. A trip to 7-Eleven was not only a time of father-daughter bonding for me, but it meant that I was guaranteed a sugary Slurpee, chocolate cream donut, or ice cream sandwich of some sort –with, of course, a pack of gum so that no evidence of my sugar escapade would be obvious to my mother upon my return home.

Fast-forward twenty years and gas stations have developed into mini-superstores of luxury and choice. They are welcoming, they are brightly lit, they have everything and anything a sweet or salty (or alcoholic) tooth could crave – available in the time it takes you to pump your gas. It is as if America preaches instant gratification around every turn of the highway. The theme is hard to avoid, impossible to run from, and like sinking sand; once you give in, it is hard to break free.

We are the land of the free, but we are a nation enslaved to food and to instant gratification. People tend to either recognize this fact or deny it. Being the all-or-nothing society that we are, we have a tendency to take things to extremities. My clients are typically either obsessed with learning about food and their daily fat and calorie intake, or they are the opposite of the spectrum completely: they make a distinct effort to not care. My clients only reiterate the reoccurring theme that balance in America is nonexistent. Balance and freedom are very difficult to find in our nation's relationship with food.

Whether our obsession with food is expressed by over-indulging or by starving ourselves, our society has created a world of contradictions. We preach freedom and individuality, yet we obsess over Hollywood and imitate celebrities. We are one of the wealthiest countries in the world, but the rich are getting richer and the poor are getting poorer. We have access to an incredible amount of natural resources, yet we are one of the highest polluting countries in the world. We have the best health clubs in the world, the largest number of personal trainers, and long stretches of farmland to provide the freshest, healthiest food we could possibly need. Yet we are the fattest country in the world. We worship athletes, sports and competitions, but unfortunately, it the number of sports bars that is growing rather than active participants in sports.

We are a nation that loves easy fixes. The ever-growing industry of diet pills alone indicates the desperation we feel. Just take two pills three times a day and you will finally achieve a flat stomach! Walk into a GNC or Vitamin Shoppe and you will discover an entire section devoted to diet solutions and pills promising to boost your natural fat metabolic rate.

If it is it easy, it does not work. Taking a pill will not get you the perfect body. Most of the diet pills on the market are not FDA approved and have been known to render terrible side effects, including headaches, nausea, heart palpitations, shakiness, diarrhea and insomnia. On top of it all, these pills over-stimulate our endocrine system and our body starts to shut down in response to the foreign substance that throws off its natural balance. When even the physiology of our bodies demands balance – from our internal pH levels, to sleep needs, to exercise and rest needed – it's time we take the hint.

It seems that the more money we invest on changing our appearance, the more dissatisfied we become. Think about the growing popularity of plastic surgery – breast augmentation, stomach tucks, calf implants, butt implants and liposuction. I have worked with a client in the past that had multiple cosmetic surgeries, bi-monthly Botox treatments, and liposuction on multiple sections of her 135 lbs. frame. She struggles daily in accepting her body and seeks my opinion consistently as to whether or not I think she should pay for another liposuction surgery in order to fully rid herself the cellulite on her thighs. The more perfectly she shapes her body through workouts and obsessive dieting, the more self-critical and harsh she becomes. My client is stuck in a never-ending hamster wheel of finding happiness through a perfect physique.

Why are we convinced that physical perfection guarantees happiness? Whatever happened to the real pursuit of happiness?

The health club industry is not exempt from the false advertising of an easy fix. Notorious for iron-clad contracts and cancellation policies, health clubs entice folks who simply want to take a more proactive step to toning up and getting healthy. This does vary from gym to gym and club to club, but unfortunately most Americans who are taking the first step into fitness never get the emotional support, direction and encouragement that they need to truly succeed in their journey. They end up giving up after a few weeks and resign to being "stuck" in the body they are in.

The fitness industry is one of the most successful, growing businesses in the market. Every day, people join by the hundreds and thousands. Simultaneously, paying members stop using the gym by the hundreds and thousands because life just gets too busy for them to make it to the gym.

Unfortunately, approximately 85% of those who join a gym never see results from their hours of sweating to the oldies. It is not for lack of effort that they are not succeeding, but rather for lack of knowledge. It all goes back to balance. You can work out for five hours a day, but if your nutrition isn't right, your body will never change. You can have great nutrition and work out consistently, but if you are overly stressed and deprived of sleep, your hormones are unbalanced and will cause you to gain weight.

We are all so desperate to change our bodies that we want to take the fast track so that it is done and over quickly. It's not our fault; we live in a culture where we can often demand instant gratification and get it, so naturally we do the same with our bodies in our approach to the gym and dieting.

Changing your body demands a lifestyle change. A total lifestyle change that balances the elements of your life will help you make long-lasting, healthy changes. You will be amazed at how much easier and more enjoyable this approach to fitness and health is.

The role of balance cannot be overestimated in the health of a human being.

Balance is all about priorities and understanding the implications that those priorities can have on your life. I have a few weight-loss clients who have recently decided to terminate their gym membership due to financial constraint or busy schedules. They can afford to dine out at restaurants five nights a week and eat fast food at least once a day, but cannot find the ability to prioritize their physical health. Or, in planning where they spend time, they value everything in their life over the health of their own bodies. What they do not realize is that your body is your vehicle for life, and it is the only one you get. Without a healthy body, living life isn't living; it's just surviving.

Spending time on your fitness on daily basis is like maintaining a car. It is investing and caring about your future and your ability to do the things you love, to feel fully alive in your skin and to be emotionally and physically available for those you love. The lack of education and understanding of balance in America is heartbreaking, for we are truly making life harder for ourselves. Without balanced health, we are missing out on so much *joie* and potential in our lives.

Incorporating balance into your life might demand some drastic changes and, understandably, that can be scary. Committing yourself to a change in any element of your life is a serious commitment. Change is scary; it is a natural reaction and it is even more intimidating when we don't know who we truly are or who we potentially can be. It is like author C.S. Lewis penned: "…infinite joy is offered to us, like an ignorant child who wants to go on making mud pies in a slum because he cannot imagine what is meant by the offer of a holiday at the sea. We are far too easily pleased."

The reason that the majority of gym members don't eventually achieve their ultimate physical perfection is simply because they never make a full lifestyle change. It is not the gym's fault. The fault lies in lack of education and balance in society.

I tell my clients that one hour in the gym cannot make up for twenty-three hours of negligence. I could give anyone the workout of their life for an hour, and then, once they walk out of those gym doors, they have twenty-three hours to negate every ounce of sweat and progress that they just made.

Success in health and fitness is attained solely through a balanced approach to food and nutrition. Americans must break the cycle of making food and thinness our goals. Our state of unhealthiness is a direct reflection of our warped perception of food and our inability to live balanced daily lives. It is time for change.

AMERICA IS FAST-PACED
Skinny, Sexy à la carte
Trop de hate nuit.
[Haste makes waste.]

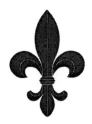

i. Skinny, Sexy SUMMARY:

Our American lives of fast food and our non-stop pace of life are making us a "fast nation" on the fast track to decline. We are a nation that loves quick fixes and instant gratification, and it seems that we have forgotten the pleasure that comes in slow living.

ii. Skinny, Sexy REFLECTION:

How scheduled is your day? *Do you ever have time during the week to spend 15 minutes over coffee with a friend?* Do you thrive of chaos or do you secretly wish that you could just catch your breath and catch a break? *What petits plaisirs in your life do you most value?* Do you get enough of these *petits plaisirs* during the week, or only on the weekend?

iii. Skinny, Sexy PERSONAL APPLICATION:

Use the time tracking chart listed in this chapter to determine how much free time you currently have and what areas of your life you might be unhappily over-committed to. Remember, we only get one life to live – and time is our most precious resource. Spend yours wisely and exactly where you want to. Even making a few small changes will transform how you feel, will make you feel empowered to pursue pleasure in life, and will dramatically minimize your stress levels.

iv. Skinny, Sexy EATING:

Experiment with natural eating for two full days. Buy nothing pre-made, "fast", processed, or with more than three ingredients listed. During these two days, sit down at a table to eat. Take your time. Make your meal or snack last you twice as long as it normally would to eat, and see how this makes you feel. Also, make a commitment to never eat in your car again.

v. Skinny, Sexy YOU:

Let go of your to-do list for a day and just live. See how it feels. If you can't completely get rid of your list, or perhaps if you absolutely love list making (which, ironically, I do), then just try to keep your list small and manageable.

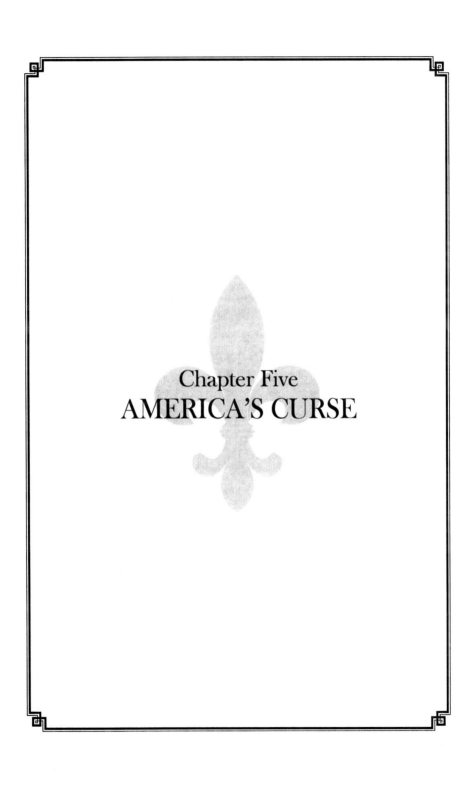

Chapter Five
AMERICA'S CURSE

Chapter Five
AMERICA'S CURSE

Over the past decade, the obesity epidemic has insidiously slipped its way into American culture and society in ways never anticipated. With adult obesity rates over 25% in many states and with over 12 million children and adolescents considered obese, the state of fatness of our nation has quickly become one of the most threatening problems for America's future. The lifestyle of inactivity, convenience and "fast" food that leads to obesity is destroying America from our youngest to our oldest and the longevity of our children's future is beginning to look bleak. We have become our own curse. Dr. Jeffrey Levi, executive director of the Trust for America's Health (TFAH) believes that "obesity is one of the biggest public health challenges the country has ever faced, and (that) troubling disparities exist based on race, ethnicity, region, and income." Levi notes that "millions of Americans still face barriers – like the high cost of healthy foods and lack of access to safe places to be physically active."

America's curse is that we are so busy in our on-the-go American lifestyle of convenience that we do not know how to properly listen to our bodies and our bodies' needs. We are either too busy to notice, or too skewed in our perceptions to figure out how to balance and prioritize our health and fitness. We sit more, walk less and spend more time in our car alone on our commutes to work than with our family and friends. If we learn to listen to our bodies, we will also learn to listen to our own souls and will begin living the way we were made to live.

It is imperative that you learn to love your body enough to respect it with the care and attention it needs. It is time you stop putting forth effort simply to maintain a façade, and instead actually start caring. You will thrive physically and emotionally from learning to love and care for yourself. So, what do you have to lose? Freeing yourself from America's curse means that you must alter your view of health and fitness. Rather than seeing it as a chore, let it become a part of the joy of living. This, my friend, is the beginning of *a skinny mind*.

We struggle to give up processed food and unhealthy eating patterns mostly because it involves great effort and an all-encompassing lifestyle change. We are gluttons for convenience. For many, our self-confidence is so low that we are afraid to risk putting any effort into changing because ultimately, we are more afraid of failure. And if we commit ourselves to health and still ultimately fail, then where is our worth? We are a nation terribly afraid of failure because we are desperately caught up in achievement-based worth.

The American lifestyle has also been blinded by mass advertising and convenience packaging. We have been hoodwinked by or own culture and success. We are so obsessed with success that we are like a prisoner to cupid's arrow, unaware of our predicament and naively seeking attention from anyone who will love us. People under cupid's arrow are blinded by love. They have lost themselves and are weak and predictable. The deeper in love you are, the foggier your vision becomes. The same is seen when we fall prey to society's praises, a fast food lifestyle, or on-the-go multi-tasking. We become so numb to the pace of our lives and the unhealthiness we invoke upon our bodies, that we are blind to the real life that we are missing out on.

We are risking our true lives in the midst of the American curse of busyness. In turn, we need to embrace the risk of "slowing down" in order to save ourselves. To properly slow down your life, you may have to cut out some things in your daily schedule, but that is where the risk lies. Will you allow yourself to slow down and be still? It is not until you are still and alone with yourself that your mind is free to really understand and analyze what you actually love in life. Living without the element of risk that comes from embracing any kind of change, is no life at all. In most situations, a person must choose to take a risk, or forever regret that chance. Do not allow yourself to lose your chance to change your life.

Anyone who has been in love can attest to the fact that regardless of how the relationship ended, love is always worth the risk. To love and be loved, no matter how painfully it may have ended, is better than never having loved at all. Fitness and living life to the fullest can be viewed the same. *Taking your life to the next level involves making proactive choices, making changes, and embracing the risk that comes with adding new elements to your life.*

People often fear or put off exercise because of the pain, the discipline, and the commitment it demands. We are often overwhelmed by the daunting feat exercise can seem to be and so we make excuses, or we commit temporarily for a month or two, but never fully or with our whole hearts. If you are unable to make a caring commitment to your health, then you are not at the point of understanding the essential role that a healthy body and body image play in your life. Exercise is a state of mentality. The more you think of exercise as play time and as simply moving your body, the less it will feel like work and the easier it will be to commit. Everyone can enjoy exercise –you simply have to find what you like and stick with it.

Emulate the freedom seen in the French culture and start taking risks to follow the things in your heart that make you tick. Take a risk, and know you lived life to the fullest, or live in fear and regret never having taken a chance. If you are not making mistakes in life, then you are not trying hard enough.

Modern America is afraid to sweat and this is what sets us apart from the French, who hate to sweat. America was built on sweat, blood and the courage of risk-takers. How, then, did we lose something that was so intrinsic to our history?

Your opportunity to break free, to fight the past decades of lifestyle degradation and stand for change that matters lies in your very own hands. The decision to take the risk of truly living, of *joie de vivre*, is your choice.

America's curse is also that we are so accustomed to dieting and so culturally inundated by the multibillion dollar diet industry that we don't know how to be healthy naturally. Instead of returning to nature by eating a French or Mediterranean diet of balance and real food, we feed our bodies over-processed chemical combinations that we have convinced ourselves is food. We spend billions on diet pills, trendy detoxifying cleanses, health club memberships and frozen diet dinners and yet we are getting fatter and fatter as a nation with every passing year.

While in France, I rarely heard the word diet, or *régime* as the French would say. Catherine Saint-Jean, my host mother in Tours, was actually a professional cook and her husband Yves was a locally renowned author and artist. Every night *chez le Saint-Jeans* we feasted on a multi-course meal, typically comprised of Catherine's recipes that Yves had published in his most recent cookbook. Catherine was serious about food and about teaching her foreign boarders a thing or two about it during their stay.

In the Saint-Jean household, where up to twelve foreign students would lodge, Catherine shopped the *marché* on a daily basis. She bought only what she could carry, and it was the perfect amount to feed the family of fifteen that she cared for. It never occurred to her that she could purchase a lot of food at one time and store it. She knew that if she did the freshness and taste of what she presented would be compromised and that is something she would never risk. The only foods she kept an abundance of were fruit and Nutella, as those were the available snacks and breakfasts that her students were allowed to have at any time.

On Sunday afternoons, Catherine held weekly cooking lessons for her lodgers, instructing us carefully, like a magician orchestrating a miraculous trick, changing simple ingredients into a food masterpiece. After a few weeks of sessions, she would "graduate" us with a mini ceremony and a certificate hand painted by Yves, appropriately coined the *Forchette d'or*, or Golden Fork.

Living with the Saint-Jeans was a curse that turned into a blessing for my body image. I loved my host family and, for Catherine, I had to express that love by being excited about food and by eating everything she offered me. She refused to let any student leave the house for class without breakfast and she always sent us off with fruit in our hand for a snack.

I was petrified the first two weeks to eat anything she offered, as I couldn't identify most of it and the only thing I could identify were the oils and fats she used to cook them. After I started to get hungry and realize that I was missing out on culture, I began tasting everything I was offered. A few weeks later, once I realized I had not gained any weight, I began tasting even more, and every now and again taking seconds. I was praised and coddled endlessly by Catherine when I ate heartedly. We would sit together for family dinner, *en famille* as French culture dictates, fifteen of us around the table, and spend an hour and a half passing the soup, main course, salad, cheese, fruit and dessert.

It was in those hours spent at the table in Tours that I experienced freedom from calorie counting for the first time. The Saint-Jeans forced me to eat breakfast and regular meals. Catherine displayed such love through gastronomy that it forced me to reconsider the role of food in my life. Previous to those dinners with Yves and

Catherine, food was simply food. The Saint-Jeans taught me the profound lesson that food was a wonderful social connector and family recharger. In Catherine's cooking lessons, she taught me to play with chocolate and feel like a child again, tasting sugar. I have never seen food the same since.

The accessibility of food in America has warped our society's understanding of food. Food is so available, no matter where we are, that we have lost value in creating a social atmosphere around food the way it is experienced in France. Americans eat while driving, watching TV, pumping gas, and traveling via public transportation. The average American's diet is heavy with carbohydrates and synthetically processed food, which acidifies after digestion. For optimal health, the body's internal pH must be balanced, but the bulk of the American diet has us overloading on acidity on our pH scale. An overly acidic internal environment causes disease and internal imbalance, which offsets the proper performance of many bodily functions.

Our nation needs a food cleanse; we need fresh fruits and vegetables to be more affordable and more available. We need safer community walking areas, playgrounds, bike paths and tools to enable us to become a more ambulatory nation. Also, we need a cleansing from our over-powering desire for financial success; we need to learn that success is relative and the most meaningful, fulfilling successes in life often do not have anything to do with a bigger house, larger SUV or more expensive dinner out. If we can redefine and reprogram what type of "success" will bring us happiness, then we will start to break free from the societal curse that holds us back.

In America, our success is, in a way, our curse. The more we succeed, the more we are driven towards perfectionism, the pursuit of money, and the approval of others. In many ways, we are living against our own nature. We are living against the founding nature of our county which is based in freedom, because we have enslaved ourselves to the opinions of others to define our success and happiness.

If you begin to define your identity or worth as a human being on your professional or financial success, then you are falling under the curse and you will never have a *skinny, sexy mind* or *joie de vivre*. Our nation's state of our health, both physical and mental, is deteriorating annually, mostly because we are not focused on the right things in life to bring us happiness.

AMERICA'S CURSE
Skinny, Sexy *à la carte*
Suffisance vaut abundance.
[Enough is as good as a feast.]

i. Skinny, Sexy SUMMARY

America's curse is that we are so busy in our on-the-go American lifestyle of convenience that we do not know how to properly listen to our bodies and our bodies' needs. We are either too busy to notice, or too skewed in our perceptions to figure out how to balance and prioritize our health and fitness.

ii. Skinny, Sexy REFLECTION:

What do you have to lose if you alter your current state of health? *How would your life change if you had time to slow down and breathe?* Do you feel like you are a slave to your over-booked schedule and that you will never be done? *Will you allow yourself to slow down and be still?*

Life, without an element of risk and change is not life at all. How does change make you feel? *Excited?* Empowered? *Scared?*

iii. Skinny, Sexy PRACTICAL APPLICATION:

Taking your life to the next level involves making proactive choices, making changes, and embracing the risk that comes with adding new elements to your life. Are you ready and willing to make these proactive, life-changing choices? You can start making changes in your life by learning more about yourself and about what makes you tick. Do something "risky" to help figure this out and see how it feels.

iv. Skinny, Sexy EATING:

Eliminate the word "diet" from your vocabulary. The first three letters of the word are "die," so it's no wonder that diets make us all feel and live miserably. Instead of dieting, think about eating whole, healthy foods. Shop at your weekly local farmer's market and look into joining a local "slow food movement."

v. Skinny, Sexy YOU

Commit to eating once a week *en famille* and start celebrating how food brings loved ones together. Be aware of healthy calories versus empty calories, but grant yourself freedom from calorie obsession. Stop yourself when you catch yourself striving for anyone else's approval other than your own.

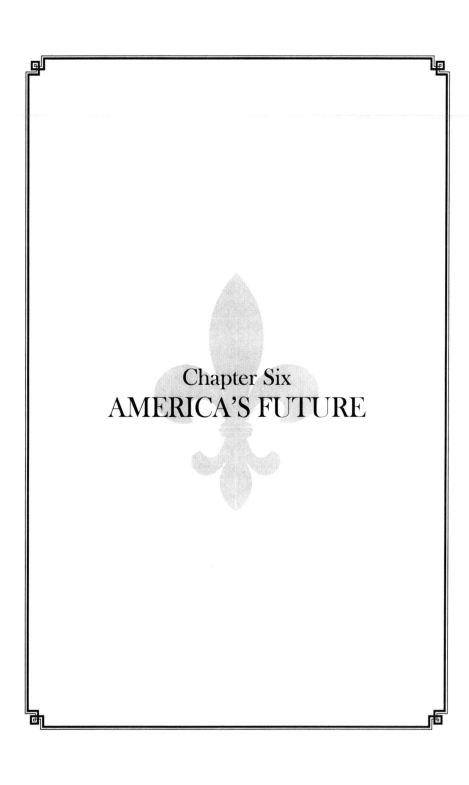

Chapter Six
AMERICA'S FUTURE

Chapter Six
AMERICA'S FUTURE

The future of American society is currently swaying in the wind; what happens in the social development of our great nation over the next decade will determine the real prognosis.

We are teetering between a generation of anorexics and a generation of bulimics and we have produced the first generation in decades that is expected to have a shorter life expectancy than their parents. The danger our children are in must be recognized and addressed, but first it must be understood.

A girlfriend of mine who works as a nanny has given me insight into the insidious nature of this epidemic. The three children she babysits are wonderfully behaved, very intelligent and sweet. However, they are extremely out of shape and overweight. My friend struggles to convince them to be active, to go outside to ride their bikes, and to play simply for the sake of playing. They don't want to play outside, they want to play video games or be on Facebook. Kids have been conditioned to expect rewards for everything, and being outside is not a reward anymore.

Don't blame parenting, TV, or the school system – in this case it has nothing to do with any of those factors – rather, it is a societal development and a generational change that cannot be attributed to just one institution.

I became all the more aware of this change in America after I moved back from France. Out of the approximately two hundred French children I taught, I can only recall a mere half a dozen that would be considered overweight. Out of those six children, only two were classifiable as clinically obese.

I moved back to American in June 2006 and spent much of the summer lifeguarding at my local summer pool. Previous to that summer, I had lifeguarded for seven years. I finally noticed in 2006 that with every year that passed, the bathing suit clad children that I stared at for hours on end were becoming increasingly larger.

In fact, the biggest culture shock I faced in transitioning back to American living was the number of obese and severely overweight children that frequented the pool. It was heart wrenching to watch eight-year-olds waddling around the pool deck and breathing with difficulty. Kids rolled themselves out of the water onto the deck like beached whales instead of being able to push up and leap out like healthy kids.

While guarding, it was alarming to watch the volume of sugar, soda, chips, candy and ice cream that parents shoved into their kids' mouths to keep them out of their hair. I lifeguarded overweight kids that were given some form of candy or sugar every hour on the hour. As I sold Chipwich sandwiches to them during Adult Swim, I remembered my French students' snack time that consisted of slices of fresh bread, fruit, water, and *small* pieces of dark chocolate. My students would devour the fruit, have a few bites of bread, and take one small piece of chocolate and before scuttling off to play enthusiastically in the recess area.

Many parents are refusing to do their job. We are taking the easy way out. We are putting our children's health on the back-burner and putting them at a disadvantage socially, mentally, and physically. We are shortening the life expectancy of an entire generation through severe nutritional neglect, over-committed schedules, and the inability to say "no".

It has become socially unacceptable to consider children fat; as a society we tiptoe around self-esteem issues rather than address the basic lifestyle changes that would actually build self-esteem within a child and their health. Instead of getting these obese children the help and guidance they need, we ignore that the problem even exists and allow them to slowly start killing themselves from the inside out. We justify ourselves saying that they're just chubby and that they'll outgrow it once they hit a growth spurt. We are lying to ourselves and are shortening the life expectancy of our children.

We are raising a generation of ignorance and disease, and we are too politically correct to give these kids a fighting chance. Generation XL is a generation that have been raised without guidance. It is a generation of children who has no grasp on the value of patience, mostly because, well, neither do we. Patience is a virtue – a virtue that is becoming obsolete in America. In this great nation, we want what we want, and we want it immediately. We are taught that if we work hard we can attain anything. What is not often recognized is that hard work takes time, patience, and most importantly, it demands balance.

America is so used to fat people that we cannot even distinguish obesity among ourselves. This mentality starts at the root of our competitive society which allows and breeds us to compare ourselves to others in order to assess our value. Ironically, we are a fat-phobic culture where some people would rather die than be overweight; our fears and desires are completely confused.

Judging others physically is done by insecure people in order to build themselves up in comparison to others. In comparing yourself to others, you always lose at the end because you will never stop comparing and critiquing yourself. The point is, not all overweight individuals overeat.

We are guilty of being a society that makes inappropriate and unapologetic assumptions about those who are overweight. Someone who is two hundred pounds overweight, must, we assume, overeat and gorge themselves. We presume that if they would just stop going to McDonalds and eating Ben and Jerry's then they wouldn't be so large. Societal tendency is to judge and unfortunately we buy into it. We are too quick to judge.

Truth be told, most overweight Americans don't eat enough. Most of us don't even slow down our lives enough to realize that or to educate ourselves on what real nutrition and health can mean for our lives and happiness. It's time to start appreciating life for how it is meant to be lived – in the small details.

America raises generations to believe in the American Dream. And believe we do, but what really is the American Dream? Our ancestors believed it to be the pursuit of happiness, health, and family. Modern Americans have crafted a dream of perfection, wealth, and luxury. It is no wonder that more Americans are on anti-depressants than ever before, that our children are battling diseases that are an onset of obesity, and that the rest of our youth are killing themselves from the inside out in an effort to have the perfect body. Somewhere along the way we convinced ourselves that having a body deemed beautiful and acceptable by societal standards would bring us happiness.

General XL has a dual nature; it is also Generation XS. We have developed into a society that cares more about being skinny than being healthy. We have forgotten where we come from and what American Dream will really bring us happiness. 53% of thirteen-year-old American girls are dieting, 25% of college women have an eating disorder, and approximately 67% of American woman have an Eating Disorder Not Otherwise Specified, or an EDNOS. These aren't just statistics, these are people.

I once met with a timid, 19 year-old Guamanian beauty, with eyes as big as a doe. She sat across from me for an hour and hung her head in shame. As she started to open up to me, honesty poured out of her eyes. In our conversation, she flashed me some of the most moving, vibrant smiles I have ever seen. In her I saw so much life, so much joy, so much personality, yet all so hidden, so repressed and pushed below the surface. You see, Amber has learned, after a 3-year-long abusive relationship, to trust no one. Yet something crying out for help deep inside her allowed her to be vulnerable with me.

Amber throws her food up. She has been throwing up for over two years. She comes from a broken family. Her relationship with food rotted and disintegrated as a control response to the abuse from her boyfriend. She embarked upon the path of bulimia as a solution to her sadness. Amber made a bulimia-pact with her best friend and they convinced themselves that life would be perfect once they were skinny enough. She confessed to me that she and her friend competed on how many boxes of laxatives they went through each week and how many pounds they lost. They got attention from guys at the clubs when they went out, and were able to hide their secretive habits from everyone who knew them.

Today, Amber lives in agony. On the weekdays, she works long days and is able to sustain herself on energy drinks and black-market Adderall. Weekends are harder on her; she works her side job at a restaurant and is forced to eat because her co-workers make comments if she doesn't. She is frightened and disgusted watching Americans gorge on the all-you-can-eat buffet. Saturday and Sunday are her bulimic days; she is now able to control exactly how much she vomits, at exactly what time, and how many laxatives she needs to take to compensate for what she consumed earlier in the day. She hides from the world, and typically goes to bed at 6:00pm. She is not losing any weight, but is terrified to change her ways.

The greatest tragedy of all is that her family doesn't think she has a problem. She expressed her struggle to her father and he believes she only wants attention. Her mother is too overwhelmed with her own life to even care to listen. Amber's older sibling has agreed that maybe a gym membership would be a better idea, and that is how I came to meet her.

We have to stop living in an America of silence. We have to stop pretending that there are not thousands of Ambers out there, many of whom are lost in themselves.

When I first sought help from my family, they thought I was being melodramatic about my body image and food consumption. They struggled to understand why I couldn't just snap out of it and realize that I looked fine in the mirror. It was practically impossible for me to explain to them the unpredictable circus mirror that I looked in every day, and the agony it caused me. It took them five years to fully understand my struggle, and from that moment on they have supported me in every way possible. Often, some family members and friends don't have the tools of understanding and healing to respond in the way you want them to or in the way a professional could. It is for that reason that I encourage anyone struggling with body image, food or obsessive exercise to meet with a professional counselor with a specialization in eating disorders.

I urge you to help break the silence. We have to start asking our daughters, our sons, our friends, and our loved ones if they struggle with their body image or their relationship with food if we suspect that they are developing unhealthy patterns. And when they answer us, we have to believe what they say. The future of our loved ones and our nation depends upon helping the millions of people who have lost their voice on their inexorable quest for physical perfection.

These conversations must be had. Our nation is desperate for dialogue on what is really going on so that anorexia, bulimia, binging and all other eating disorders not otherwise specified can be discussed. We need to shine some light into the darkness of the 30+ million Americans who silently struggle in shame with their body, food, and self-worth.

It is our human obligation to support the countless souls who hate the skin they are in and to show them that there is a healthy, easier, and happier way to live. We *can* put an end to the silence, to the humiliation, to the judgment and we do that by starting to help. If you know someone who needs your help, the most important thing to do is to listen. Listen, and then ask questions. Encourage the person you are worried about to seek professional help and affirm in them that they are not alone in their struggle. Remind them that there is nothing to be ashamed of, either in having an eating disorder, or in seeking counsel, and applaud them for having the courage to want to change.

I recently received an email plea from a 40-year-old mother. Loretta described herself as low-income and desperate for change. A single mother of three, she weighs over three hundred pounds. Loretta works a full-time job on her feet and due to the strain of her body frame, is having debilitating hip and knee pain that makes it extremely difficult to walk and move. Right now, Loretta lives on her minimum wage job and governmental assistance and cannot afford a gym membership, healthy groceries or her own transportation.

Loretta is begging for help, and she doesn't know where to turn. She has found that she can feed her family the cheapest and easiest from local fast food dollar menus and frozen dinners. When she and I discussed daily caloric consumption, she had no idea what a calorie was and how it impacted her body.

Loretta is hungry for knowledge. It is not a diet that will save Loretta and her family; it is education on nutrition, exercise, balance and health.

Help is at our very fingertips if we start loving and educating ourselves and others more. Love will cascade into self-acceptance. Self-acceptance will inspire individual freedom and knowledge will prevail. We have to stop caring about what everyone else is doing, what everyone else looks like, and how much money everyone else makes, and remember that the those are not things that will bring us happiness in life. Happiness comes in finding contentment and confidence in your own body and inner identity so that you can live carefree and able to relish in life's simple pleasures.

It's time to be vocal and it's time to ask the tough questions.

The worst aspect of an eating disorder is the loneliness. I spent years thinking that I was a freak and was the only one struggling with such a turbulent body image. When consumed by food or self-image, there is so much internal shame involved that sufferers are very unlikely to seek out help themselves. If we want the people we love to be vocal, we are going to have to help them along the way and make them realize that they are not alone in this. If you are fighting to love the skin you are in, rest assured that you are not alone and you can break free. Begin by removing the things and people in your life that bring you down: friends who obsessively talk about their weight and appearance, the scale in your bathroom and your subscription to Cosmo Magazine. Whatever it is that holds your mind in constant focus on your physical appearance, flee that and focus on something outside of you and your own insecurities. The following are some thought-provoking questions to consider for yourself or for someone you love; talk about your answers with someone and start breaking the silence. I promise it will feel good.

SAVING AMERICA'S FUTURE

SAMPLE QUESTIONS TO ASK SOMEONE STRUGGLING WITH BODY IMAGE

- How can I help?

- How often do you think about food or count calories?

- What are your fears about your body, your weight, and about how others perceive you?

- Do you define your worth as a human being based on the number on the scale?

- Have you ever turned down an invitation to go out with friends because you felt fat that day?

- How closely do you read nutrition labels?

- Are you afraid to eat food with fat in it?

- Are you afraid to eat carbohydrates?

- Are you meticulous in counting grams of sugar?

- Do you ever eat because you are depressed?

- Do you eat when you are bored and then feel guilty later?

- Would you rather be fat or have a terminal illness?

- How many times a day do you eat?

- Do you ever intentionally skip meals?

- Do you ever feel guilty after eating?

- Do you ever over-eat, or binge, and then purge?

- When you exercise, do you ever feel like you are exercising specifically to make up for something you ate?

- Have you ever eaten so much that you have intentionally made yourself sick?

- Do you get nervous to look in the mirror or at pictures?

- How do you feel about yourself if you see an unflattering picture?

- Do you avoid mirrors and pictures?

- Do you weigh yourself more than once a week?

- If you weigh heavier than you would like, how does that number on the scale make you feel? Does it cause you anxiety?

- What three things do you love about your body?

- Are there parts of your body that you hate and think about constantly?

- Have you ever been ashamed about something you ate?

- Does the thought of putting on a bathing suit make you anxious?

- Do you avoid intimacy unless it is dark?

- Do you constantly compare your body to others?

- Have you ever thought you would finally be happy if you just lost ten pounds?

There is, in my opinion, no more beautiful way to articulate self-confidence than with the French phrase for confidence *bien dans sa peau*, which, quite literally translates to "being well in one's skin." Neither "self-esteem," nor "positive self-image" suits a concept so well as *bien dans sa peau*. What more could one want than to be fully comfortable in the skin you are born in?

Here is my challenge to you: love the skin you are in. Love it today. Love it with no exceptions. It is a challenge that I preach to every one of my clients, and it changes lives.

One by one we can start a revolution of change. We must. It is by one person at a time that we change the world. It will be one skin at a time that we will change the well-being and balance of the American lifestyle. America's future is at stake – will you take part in the solution?

FINDING *Joie de Vivre* IN FOOD

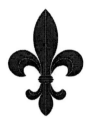

- Sit down while you eat.

- Eat with someone else and talk about the tastes.

- Chew slowly and take your time.

- Do not eat fast food. There is nothing healthy about it.

- Eat breakfast; the French never skip it.

- Allow yourself small splurges that you love, but keep them small.

- Everything in moderation is OK.

- Never eat until you are full, eat until you are satisfied.

- Eat something green every time you eat.

- Never skip meals; it will slow down your metabolism.

- Have a dinner party with friends. Try to make it last three hours.

- Eat fresh fruit, locally farmed meats, wild fish and organic vegetables.

- Do not add salt or sugar to anything. Too much salt and sugar damage your taste buds and your ability to enjoy a plethora of tastes.

- Try a new food every week to keep your taste palate always exploring and developing.

AMERICA'S FUTURE
Skinny, Sexy à la carte
Plaie d'argent n'est pas mortelle..
[Money isn't everything.]

i. Skinny, Sexy SUMMARY

We are teetering between a generation of anorexics and a generation of bulimics and we have produced the first generation in decades that is expected to have a shorter life expectancy than their parents. The danger our children are in must be recognized and addressed, but first it must be understood.

ii. Skinny, Sexy REFLECTION:

It is our human obligation to support the countless souls who hate the skin they are in and to show them that there is a healthy, easier, and happier way to live. We can put an end to the silence, to the humiliation, to the judgment and we do that by starting to help. How are you helping?

Are you ready to have the hard to have conversations with yourself and/or with those you love?

Are you setting a positive example for others in your life?

iii. Skinny, Sexy PERSONAL APPLICATION:

This is the challenge before America: love the skin you are in. Love it today. Love it with no exceptions. Are you willing to take on this challenge?

iv. *Skinny, Sexy EATING*

Get your body fat tested by a local certified personal trainer or health professional. Ask advice on what your optimal healthy body weight should be based on your height and fitness level. Remember that more often than not, our weight goals are twisted and made extreme due to cultural influence, so seeking professional advice on what really is your healthy happy weight is essential information.

v. *Skinny, Sexy YOU*

Be honest with yourself and others about these hard questions. Reach out to those around you and create community.

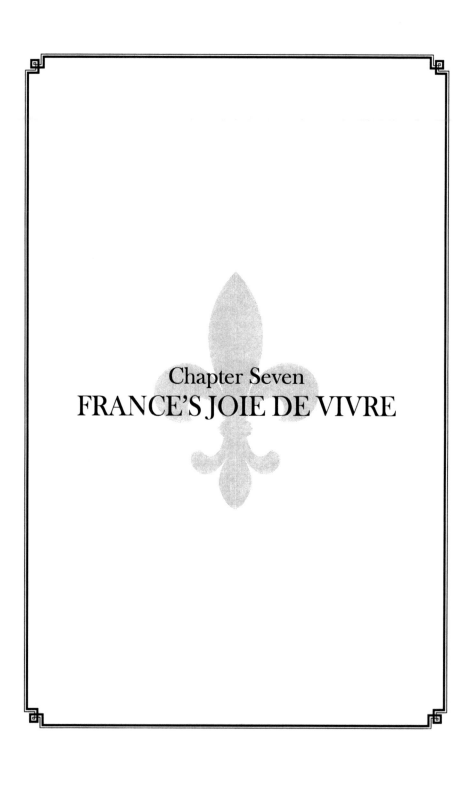

Chapter Seven

FRANCE'S JOIE DE VIVRE

Chapter Seven
FRANCE'S JOIE DE VIVRE

One of the most influential elements of French society that can be incorporated into our American lives is the concept of *joie de vivre*. *Joie de vivre* literally translates as "joy for living," but the concept encompasses so much more. *Joie de vivre* is a buoyant enjoyment of life and a keen delight in being alive. In realigning the mind to have this concept at the forefront of life, we naturally begin to allow our splendid uniqueness to shine in the world.

Joie de vivre is French society's way of recognizing that life is short and must be appreciated for its wonder, joys, sorrows and mysteries. It is *carpe diem* that they actually live out. We too can embrace *joie de vivre*; once we begin to see that by focusing on simplicity of mind and balance in life, pleasure will ripple throughout our lives farther than we can possibly imagine. Once you experience *joie de vivre*, you will never turn back to your complicated life of to-do lists.

I regret to admit that most Americans, myself included, are often so preoccupied with making money and being successful in the eyes of others that we forget some of the basic principles for good, healthy, happy living. Our nation was founded upon the idea of the pursuit of happiness; unfortunately, we just pursued it in the wrong direction.

What would happen if every day, every American connected with their *joie de vivre*? Laughter would cushion each daily activity; mundane jobs would become vibrant opportunities, Monday mornings would be looked forward to, and the rising depression rate among Americans would plummet. Most of us simply fluff our days with activities, with obligations and with errands. We do so because we are told to. As children we are taught the American way to succeed financially and we do our very best to stick to the tried-and-true beaten path of our predecessors. We live fast-paced and over-committed. Many of us keep ourselves so non-stop busy that we don't realize that, despite all our efforts to fluff them up, we actually have no fill to our lives.

Experiencing France made me see that I could live my life as a gift, not a to-do list. You can, too.

The French fill their lives with *joie de vivre.* Every Epicurean aspect of French cuisine, every probing query of philosophical exploration, every stitch of Parisian couture and dinner *soirée* of endless wine and cheese all equally reflect the same image: *joie.* This *joie* is grounded in a deep national intimacy of sharing of the human experience. It is an understanding that the human experience should be lived in awe and appreciation, and that while life has certain tragedies and difficulties, we are made to cherish the small things in life to experience living and survive the bad.

Stephen Clarke, bestselling author of *A Year in the Merde* and *Talk to the Snail: Ten Commandments For Understanding the French* has a firm grasp on France's relationship with food. He asserts: "You can't live in France if you're not interested in food. The French do not respect people who deny themselves any pleasure at all, and, despite what they might try to tell the world, they take food even more seriously than sex." He also notes the importance of seasonal, fresh and regional foods and ingredients in the French diet. Farmers markets do not have to be advertised, nor are they special events. They are the crux of society. Every Saturday and Wednesday in any small town across France you can expect the cobblestone streets to be jammed with shoppers, lists in hand, choosing their fruits and vegetables with artistry in preparation for their *menu fixe* planned for that evening..

Philosophy is at the heart of France; natives are intrinsically proud of their existentialist ancestors and aspire to think as profoundly for themselves. Discovering your *raison d'être* and your *joie de vivre* is your ticket to being one step closer to philosophers like Rousseau, Descartes and Sartre. It is all about you; you are the only thing that matters and, at the end of the day, there is really no set uniform purpose to living. The purpose of living therefore depends upon what brings *you* pleasure. We were all created to enjoy different things, so enjoy what you love, for you were made for that. Live with all your might and live to maximize the *joie* and beauty you can experience in your daily living.

ACTIVITIES THAT FILL ME WITH *JOIE:*

- I Enjoy: _____

  _____

- Five Reasons Why I Enjoy It: _____

  _____

- I Enjoy: _____

  _____

- Five Reasons Why I Enjoy It: _____

  _____

- I Enjoy: _____

  _____

- Five Reasons Why I Enjoy It: _____

  _____

- I Enjoy: _____

  _____

- Five Reasons Why I Enjoy It: _____

  _____

- I Enjoy: _____

  _____

- Five Reasons Why I Enjoy It: _____

  _____

The first step of living with *joie* in France begins with food. It must be understood that the French relish in every aspect of Epicurean delight: in the texture, freshness, spice selection, and presentation of food. Typically, when thinking of American pleasure associated with food, we envision sugary or butter-laden dishes. The French differ from America in that they are raised with a cultural appreciation for a healthy dietary balance; they have been surrounded by it from their earliest days of childhood spent playing among vegetable stands in the streets while their parents meticulously shopped the *Marché*. Pleasure is found in balance. Clarke describes a brilliant example of the ingrained importance of balance, despite the Americanization of France:

> ...amidst the chocolate cakes and buttery tarts, healthy eating is high on the menu. A cheese or ham sandwich will probably be *aux crudités* – with lettuce and tomato – and will have one slice of cheese rather than the four that are stuffed into an American sandwich.[...] So yes, like all the developed nations, the French are getting fatter. But they are doing so less quickly, because most of them just aren't interested in eating processed garbage instead of balanced meals.

Even though I describe decadent French dinner parties and luxurious seaside breakfasts of white wine, croissants and oysters, never once was the total portion size of the meals near the size of what an average American meal from a restaurant looks like. The French understand balance, and for them, that begins in portion sizes. Even Starbucks Coffee stores in France serve smaller sized coffee and pastries. They do not have a *Venti* cup size and all pastries are about half the size of what you find in American stores. A French person would have no need for a 20 ounce *Venti* coffee and understands that consuming something in such a large quantity is both wasteful and unhealthy for the body. Multi-course meals can have up to eight courses, but each one is small and delicate, allowing the diner to slow down while eating, to taste and savor the flavor combinations and food presentation. Moreover, courses are spread out in between conversation, allowing the stomach to digest and for diners to cleanse their palates in order to fully enjoy their next course. Balance is expressed in every element of French eating.

Joie de vivre also isn't found in looking a certain way. It is not found in beauty or in being beautiful, and it certainly has no correlation to being skinny or super fit. *Joie de vivre* is about exploring the depths of your own soul and living every desire with fervency and without fear. It is the innate sense of adventure woven profoundly into your human nature that your heart begs for you to embrace. *Joie de vivre* is real liberty in every sense of the word. It is not something that can be forced; rather it must be felt, lived out, and experienced.

In many ways, I believe that *joie* is the ability to let go of perfectionism. Perfectionism is a trait common in the United States among those of us desperate to succeed by societal standards and to receive approval from others. Whether it be perfectionism in one's body, in raising perfect children, in athletics, in moving up along the corporate ladder or simply in housekeeping, perfectionism typically ends in personal catastrophe. Striving for perfection is actually limiting; in doing so, you are seeking to achieve unattainable limits that are set and controlled by others. Your inflexible attitude will result in personal devastation and constant frustration. Moreover, perfectionism always leads to self-criticism, and self-criticism is deadly for *joie de vivre*.

Taoist principles on self-criticism and the role of the mind echo the concept of *joie*. In the Tao I Ching no.27 there is a saying that reflects the French practice of upholding *joie de vivre*. The Tao says: "You should exercise unrelenting discipline over your thought patterns. Cultivate only productive attitudes…You are the product of everything you put into your body and mind."

Essentially, this powerful statement of Eastern thought reminds us that our lives will mirror our thought life. In order to have the mind power to cultivate *joie,* as the Tao suggests, you have to first know and own the positive qualities that enable you to be filled with *joie.*

By constantly charging our minds with affirmations of love, we will become more in tune and empowered by our positive qualities. First however, we need to identify our positive qualities so that we can combat moments of self-criticism by our affirmations.

On the following page, come up with seven adjectives and attributes for each category. In the future, you will be able to take your attributes and implement them into affirmations of love when bombarded by self-criticism and perfectionist tendencies. It is important that you take your time in creating your list of attributes, as the more concrete these attributes become in your mind, the more you will be able to show who you are. Remember, there is beauty and *joie* in your presence if you are able to allow yourself to be and show who you are. These attributes will help you be you.

DISCOVERING YOUR PERSONAL ATTRIBUTES

- My Physical Attributes Are: _____

_____

_____

- My Spiritual Attributes Are: _____

_____

_____

- My Intellectual and Professional Attributes Are: _____

_____

- My Emotional Attributes Are:_____

- My Social Attributes Are:_____

- My Personality Attributes Are:_____

First impressions – the first three to seven seconds of meeting or seeing someone – will always distinguish those with joie and those without. It is written on their face, it comes through in their smile; it sparkles in their eyes and resounds in their laughter. True *joie* is a pheromone-esque charm that touches every passer-by, every observer and every interaction. On average, our subconscious makes eleven snap judgments about a person within the first seven seconds of meeting. How do you come off to others? How you come off to others depends heavily on how you come off to yourself.

Imagine how you will come off if you have frequencies of self-criticism that dominate your thought patterns. If you reinforce your mind with affirmations of love, you will find that you will experience a sense of peace, and almost relief. *These affirmations of love essentially enable you to give yourself permission to be yourself.* If you are relaxed and content in who you are, you will find yourself less harsh towards others. You will be happier, people will be more naturally drawn to you, and you will have a new ability to impact the world in ways you never were able to before. This is the power of *joie de vivre* in knowing yourself. This is *joie* living at its best. This is freedom.

Joie de vivre is a positive energy that draws both positive people and positive circumstances into one's life and enriches the life-experience. Moreover, it is the key to freedom for those who are over-consumed by body image disorders, low self-esteem, or their relationship with food.

I have a vivid memory of lingering over a mug of coffee at a local coffee shop that will always speak *joie* to me. While looking absent-mindedly out the shop window, I observed a friendship that I will never forget: two friends, racing across the parking lot to their car. Their *joie de vivre* became more and more evident with every spin of their wheelchairs spokes. A paraplegic and a cripple, I was mes-merized by their laughter; it captivated me from the other side of the large window and I myself was paralyzed in a stare.

If those of us who have struggled, or who still struggle with poor body image could, like my two mobile "friends," de-program what our brains have convinced us will bring us happiness, then we will finally find our true *joie*.

Most who have an unhealthy relationship with food and body have prescribed to the idea that once their body is "beautiful" according to media standards, they will finally feel free, genuinely desired, and fully alive. It is severely tragic how morphed our understanding of mind-body connection is. We are crippled in our understanding of what life really is and of who we really are.

If you want to discover *joie* in your life, the first step is to identify your attributes and own them. You must repeat them to yourself on a daily basis, write them down on paper as self-affirmations to remind yourself and think on them when you are trying to silence self-criti-cism and perfectionism.

Secondly, now that your mind is strong, you must build on this foundation for living by being able to find *joie* in food. Most of us can honestly say that we love food, but many of us do not fully understand how to balance the role of food in our lives so that we stop living on a diet or feeling negatively about our bodies.

Food is to be celebrated. Please note that I said food, not fake food. Our supermarkets and restaurants have been inundated with synthetically made modifications of food, and millions of Americans don't even know the difference. Real food is not chemically processed, packaged, frozen, genetically modified or fast. If it is something you can pick up in a drive-through window or it is something you can eat while you are driving, then most likely it is not "real" food.

Make eating an event and start reading labels. If it has more than five ingredients, it is probably not made from real food. If you start to mimic the French and many other European cultures like I did, you will start to find freedom and joy in what you eat and how it makes your body feel.

While the French definitely celebrate food, they eat to live rather than live to eat. It sounds a little contradictory, but it is simply that food is not their essence or their purpose. If you can change your relationship with food to realize that it is a necessary and beautiful component of our daily lives, not to be restricted but rather to be embraced, you will begin to learn how to eat to live. If you have ever been on a diet or restricted eating plan, you have probably experienced what it feels like to live to eat. When you live to eat, you spend every day looking forward to the next meal, thinking about the next meal, or obsessing over caloric consumption.

Eating to live is freedom. When you eat to live, you are free to enjoy food without restrictions. Moreover, with this mentality, you are able to see that food is simply an element of life. It is life and energy-giving and for that it is to be celebrated and shared among others. Food is one of the centers of human connection and interaction; eating to live recognizes that and celebrates it.

The third key to developing and nurturing your *joie de vivre* is found in knowing what you like to do. Now that you know who you are (by the wonderful attributes that make you *you*) and know how to celebrate food freely, you need to know what makes you tick. It's time that you know precisely what makes your heart come alive, what fills you with enthusiasm and purpose and what makes your skin tingle when you think about it or experience it.

Many of us do what we think we like to do simply because we have always done it. For example, think about a young college softball player who has played softball since she could stand. She probably thinks she loves the sport, but does she know why she loves the sport and does she actually really love it or does she do it because her identity is so deeply tied into it? In *The Purpose Driven Life*, Rick Warren asks if someone observed you without you knowing it for two days, what would they determine motivates you? Sometimes our pleasures and motivations are not what we think…

I encourage you to think about what you like to do. Now think about whether you really like to do it or whether you simply do it because you feel like you should or you feel like you always have done it or if you just want to be the *type* of person who does love those things! There is an essential difference between liking to do something and really loving it. If you want to experience the full capacity of *joie de vivre*, you will find that by letting go of the "likes" in your life and fully pursuing the "loves" in your life, your life will begin to over-flow with *joie* you never knew possible.

Use your answers from earlier in the chapter to discover which activities in you life fill you with *joie* and why. From this exercise, which of your hobbies you do really love, and which do you actually only really like? Do you love anything? If you don't know what you love right now, that's OK; it is very common. You are now at ground zero to rebuild your ability to live life to the fullest. If you don't know what you absolutely love to do, start experimenting and living new experiences, and you will soon learn what makes you come alive. The best way to discover yourself is to do something you have never done before. Many people find that travel is the best way to do this, others find themselves in music they might not have normally listened to, and still others surround themselves with animals to discover how to love and what they love.

You are now on the road to discovering your own *joie de vivre*. It is not a set formula or paved pathway; it is your unique journey. I encourage you to find *joie* in places you never thought and to dwell on the personal attributes you are composed of, for these things will inspire you. Once you discover that life is meant to be free of judgment, perfectionism and self-criticism, you will be free to live, laugh and love in whatever ways most inspire you.

Welcome to real *joie de vivre*, welcome to the beginnings of your new *skinny mind*.

FRANCE'S JOIE DE VIVRE
Skinny, Sexy *à la carte*
Une journée est perdu si l'on n'a pas ri.
[A day without laughter is a day wasted.]

i. Skinny, Sexy SUMMARY:

Joie de vivre literally translates as "joy for living," but the concept encompasses so much more. *Joie de vivre* is a buoyant enjoyment of life and a keen delight in being alive. In realigning the mind to have this concept at the forefront of life, we naturally begin to allow our splendid uniqueness to shine in the world.

ii. Skinny, Sexy REFLECTION:

What would happen if every day you connected with your true *joie de vivre?*

Joie de vivre is based on knowing yourself. How well do you actually know yourself? Are you true to yourself or do you do things or act a certain way based on what others expect of you?

iii. Skinny, Sexy PRACTICAL APPLICATION:

Pleasure is found in balance. Find three ways this week that you can implement more balance in your life.

iv. Skinny, Sexy EATING:

The secret to *joie de vivre* with eating lies in knowing how to choose smaller, more petit portion sizes. Also, food is worthy of celebration. Stop obsessing over it, denying it to yourself, or fearing it. Food is a wonderful part of life, try to start seeing it that way.

v. Skinny, Sexy YOU:

Joie de vivre is about exploring the depths of your own soul and living every desire with fervency and without fear. The root of this *joie* is found in the ability to let go of perfectionism. Perfectionism always leads to self-criticism, and self-criticism is deadly for *joie de vivre*. Moreover, perfectionism is a choice, an unnecessary one. Accept yourself. Reject perfectionism.

Chapter Eight
FRANCE IS CONFIDENT

Chapter Eight
FRANCE IS CONFIDENT

Ralph Waldo Emerson understood the value of confidence in a world where confidence and individuality are difficult to find. He famously stated that "to be yourself in a world that is constantly trying to make you something else is the greatest accomplishment." Emerson has recognized a timeless truth, and a truth that forms the crux of French society. It is time that we live by his words and in doing so we will discover confidence that we never knew possible.

The modern American woman has an unhealthy need to seek the approval of others. In many cases, it is not just a fascination, but a dependency. For many young Americans, peer-based approval is an intense need, and contributes to the epidemic spread of eating disorders and body image dysmorphia that is plaguing our nation.

Similarly, I serve as the perfect example of someone who has had to learn by trial and error how to emulate Emerson. For too many years of my life I have sought value in the praises and approval of others. Even today my *joie* disappears instantaneously the moment I allow my mind to dwell on how other people perceive my body and my beauty. I literally become mentally self-abusive. The self-loathing and criticism that flood my thoughts are so harsh and dark that I dare not utter them out loud. This comes as a surprise to many, considering that most see me as the "All-American Girl," with an extra splash of vivacity and zest. I am as confident, bubbly, and warm as they come. I have been described to have eyes that smile and a charm able to win over anyone's trust. Yet, on some days, I have a perverted grasp of what is truly meaningful in life. I forget what matters and I forget that I don't need to live my life in the way the world wants me to. My mind knows what *joie de vivre* feels like, but, surrounded by the right (or really, wrong) influences, my body becomes reluctant and cynical, which then reawakens unhealthy thought patterns from my past.

It is at those moments that self-awareness is critical. I am able to catch myself and at those moments I remember my French friends Marie-Ode and Lucie. Neither of these two women are specifically stand-out in the objective sense of beauty, but both of them are absolutely stunning in their confident nature. When I knew them in France they were so fully alive, confident in their skin, and filled with laughter and love for life that it transformed and magnified their beauty. They are the essence of women with *skinny, sexy minds*.

Marie-Ode is slightly plump, but the way in which she embraces her body makes her one of the sexiest and most confident French women I know. She is constantly reinventing herself and her style; she changes her hair color every month and buys clothes that cling to her shapely curves and that match her vibrant personality. In a country where the language is spoken softly, Marie-Ode lives loudly. Any day that I happened to pass Marie-Ode on the streets of Périgueux, it was like running into instant fun because, *joie* is contagious. *Joie de vivre* inspires life into others. When you see someone so fully comfortable with themselves, it inspires you to be the same. Being around Marie-Ode helped me realize how much there is to celebrate in life and how much more energy you have to enjoy it when you are able to free yourself from preoccupation and worries about your body image.

Lucie was my swimming teammate from Libourne. She bounced from boyfriend to boyfriend, never allowing them to define her. Lucie is pretty and slightly built and attracts unfaithful men. Knowing her innate value, she does not stand to be treated poorly, so she promptly leaves her cheating boyfriends and continues to date freely until she truly finds the type of man she deserves. She values her independence as a young working professional and despite the turnover of male suitors, never once questions herself or her worth. An average swimmer, Lucie is in her mid-twenties and still competes in the sport because she loves the water and how it makes her feel. Though she is not the fastest, she still swims because she realizes that sport is about enjoyment and health. Lucie's image is imprinted in my mind and reminds me that life lived independently can be beautifully animated. In a nation that is notorious for complaining, I never once heard Lucie complain. In a nation known for romance, I never once heard Lucie stress over her failed relationships. Lucie doesn't waste time on such thoughts, for she focuses on living, laughing, and pursuing what she enjoys.

These women are a stark contrast to many of the women I know in the United States. For example, one of my clients, Annie, struggles fundamentally with the concept of joy. Body image is of course an issue for her as well, but the deep root of her self-image struggle is found in her lack of *joie*. Fixated on success, Annie lives her life constantly stressed out and without the ability to relax. When asked what she likes to do for fun, she can't answer me.

Annie has lost sight of herself; she lives for others. She yearns for praise and approval from friends, co-workers and her boyfriend. She is driven because, she admits she wants recognition. She conceded she is miserable but is frantically stumped on how to change.

Annie is trying to get through life, just wanting to survive. Annie doesn't know a thing about living. You can't expect to experience living when you are only focused on surviving. There is a paramount difference between living and surviving. One of the contributing factors to distinguishing this difference is found in the development of self-confidence. Confidence is something that people pay to have and pay to be around. We pay for beauty products, manicures, personal trainers, hair stylists, plastic surgeons and anything else that will make us feel externally confident and beautiful. As humans, we are naturally attracted to and feel comfortable around those who are confident. Confidence can change the entire way a person looks, is perceived, and is able to inspire others around them.

The great news is that confidence is a *choice*. It is a frame of mind that one must proactively align oneself with. You are what you think, so think yourself confident. Allow me to describe an American who is the quintessential example of someone who chooses confidence. Sophie is self-proclaimed as big and beautiful. Half Latina, half Caucasian, she is 5"4' and weighs around 250 lbs. Sophie knows that she is sexy, knows that she is gorgeous, and likes her size, but admits to having to *choose* that mindset. Sophie knows she is sexy because she is wonderfully unique. She is herself in a world that tries to make her something thing else.

That is not to say that Sophie's mastery of beauty came easily. Sophie bears scars of her battle with confidence, though one would never know it; rarely does she allow herself to be so vulnerable as to admit to ever considering herself anything but fabulous. If she ever does allow you a vulnerable glimpse into her real self, then she will reveal her legs to you. The front of her right thigh bears the marks of a cutter. Sophie explains that during a moment of darkness, years prior, she had been so overwhelmed with self-hatred and anger that she took a sharp razor blade and carved the words *"you're fat"* deeply into her flesh.

The scars will remain forever, even if only faintly, but serve as a constant daily reminder to Sophie of her triumph over negative thoughts. Sophie believes that her potential in life is limited only by negative thoughts, and she trusts that her deep inner beauty shines so strongly that her outer beauty could never be affected by the number on the scale.

One person can transform your life and your view of yourself. The friends you choose in your life can make a tremendous impact, so choose them wisely. For Sophie, it was a friend in her past named Jess that taught her to embrace herself and her voluptuous curves and to deny her desire to compare her body to others. For me, it was my friendships with the people I met in France that finally opened my eyes to this freeing concept of individual body-acceptance.

Who are the people in your life that have and will make a positive impact upon your understanding of body image and body acceptance? Conversely, can you identify those that impact you negatively and who are enablers to your destructive self-criticism? It is up to you to eliminate the toxic people from your life and to surround yourself with people who inspire you to be the best version of you possible.

It is important to know that a confident woman lives from the inside out rather than the outside in; she is able to retain the little girl innocence of knowing she has limitless potential. In our faltering moments of insecurity, we find ourselves desperately trying to look into the depths of our own beauty and remember just exactly what it is that qualifies us as beautiful. When you make being beautiful an understood fact about your identity, confidence becomes much easier to hold on to.

ENJOYING GOOD THINGS TAKES CONFIDENCE

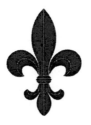

Someone once defined France itself as the capacity for enjoying good things. Enjoying good things is exactly what I learned how to do while in France, so I thoroughly agree with the statement. In fact, I like to think that the *Trépied,* the nickname for my group of three best friends, embraced such a philosophy whole-heartedly.

We learned from the best, the French themselves. A teacher that I worked for in Périgueux informed me of a French saying that transformed the way I lived the rest of my time there, and subsequently, the rest of my life so far. She said that "to be French is to be a rebel, with respect [of course] for aesthetics and beauty." A sub-thought of said philosophy is that France cultivates its past while evolving in the present, meaning that, more than anything, the present is what matters.

In France, I lived in a world where people lived without over-anticipating the future; they thrived on living in the present, a concept that is incredibly foreign to Americans. My *Trépied* comrade Angi once pointed out to me how interesting it was that in the French countryside there is a sign for every village you leave, but never a sign telling you how far away the next village is as we so often have in the States. Why anticipate the next village or the prolongation of your journey when you can simply enjoy the present moment of being in-between villages, just driving? This is a profound concept for those of us who are career and success driven, constantly on the move and looking forward to achieving happiness. *If we are always looking ahead, or looking behind, we are never really able to just look and that is where we miss out on every important and worthwhile part of real life.*

Thursdays were my favorite days of teaching in France. It was a full schedule for me, which, in French terms, meant four periods of forty minutes. Most other days were only half days, and Fridays were even better with only one class to teach in the morning. The cobblestone streets of Périgueux, population 35,000, had a life and story of its own that I discovered as I walked from school to school on my "busy" work days.

My last class on Thursdays was a group of CM2 students at La Cité, with a young teacher who wanted an English teacher primarily to give herself a daily break. My afternoons there were spent teaching 9-year-olds *Duck, Duck, Goose,* and *Ring-Around-the-Rosey* and deeming it a proper English lesson. I clapped, giggled, and played with the kids, and made sure that all words of encouragement and yells were in the token memorized English phrases: *"Go!," "Nice job!," "Awesome!,"* and *"Hurry!"*. Yes, those kids surely learned a lot of English from my lessons. Moreover, I learned that I was in no way ready for kids of my own anytime soon.

After the CM2 class, the text inbox on my cell phone would flood with messages from the *Trépied*. Caroline would message that her high school students were rebellious and had skipped their classes in order to participate in a protest against new laws on the production of *foie gras* or local taxes on wine. A *grève* (or protest), *is* an important part of national French pastime. Angi would send a SMS moan about how her snooty Portuguese roommate, who also worked with her, was driving her insane. A second group text would be exchanged stating simply: *Café de Paris. Tout de suit.*

Café de Paris, the café in Périgueux that oozed class and was quite posh for the small town where we lived. A doorman would open the entryway of the burgundy colored awning to invite us in. We would then walk into a room of café tables arranged in segmented and multilevel sections, each surrounded by plush leather burgundy couch-chairs. A long marble bar, manned by pretentious *garçons*, formed the outline of the bar boundary. Dimly lit, the entire bar resonated with sounds of jazz and classic French masterpieces. Occasionally, the sultry sounds of Norah Jones could be heard.

As Norah sang the soundtrack to our lives, we collapsed into the plush darkness in the upper rear level of the *Café de Paris*. *Café de Paris* was our oasis, our secret escape. Ironic, however, that we chose to escape the stress of our French lives in perhaps the most Parisian café atmosphere our beloved Périgueux had to offer. Something about the rigid traditionalism lured us, especially in the contradictions we felt when surrounded by the vibrantly wild individualists that would frequent the café. I liked the world of contradictions I found in France, it reminded me not to think so much and instead to just enjoy.

Vin rouge would be ordered. Fresh bread with olive oil and balsamic vinaigrette would be brought to the table. After three rounds of rouge, we would split a specialty pizza – the café's whole grain flatbread adaptation of their Italian neighbor's masterpiece. Adorned with chunks of *chèvre* and spinach, it was a pizza that could be found neither in Italy, nor in America.

Perhaps what we loved the most about *Café de Paris* was that the café itself changed us. Well, it wasn't the café, but it was the time it granted us to really absorb what it was about the French that made them so very different from us. Through the hours we spent sipping wine, watching café-goers and trying to pinpoint exactly what it was about the French that was so magnetizing, we began to embrace our own contradictory natures as well. We learned that life and time are what you make of them; stress is a choice and living well is another. We found, too, that the more you laugh, the more confident you will be. The more you laugh at your own personal contradictions, the more you will be confident in who you are and the skin you are in. And, most importantly, in that petit café in Périgueux, the French taught me that enjoying good things takes confidence.

FRANCE IS CONFIDENT
Skinny, Sexy *à la carte*
La chance sourit aux audacieux.
[Fortune favors the brave.]

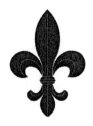

i. Skinny, Sexy SUMMARY:

Ralph Waldo Emerson famously stated that "to be yourself in a world that is constantly trying to make you something else is the greatest accomplishment." Emerson has recognized a timeless truth, and a truth that forms the crux of French society. It is time that we live by his words and in doing so we will discover confidence that we never knew possible.

ii. Skinny, Sexy REFLECTION:

What is holding you back from being confidently yourself without exception? *Have you ever felt confident in this manner, and if so, how did it feel?* What influences in your life are holding you back from being confident and true to yourself and how can you choose to tune out these negative, toxic influences?

iii. Skinny, Sexy PERSONAL APPLICATION:

Enjoying good things takes confidence. How deep is your capacity for enjoying good things? Experiment with this over a weekend; plan a weekend of wonderful outings and make a note of all of the emotions you feel as the weekend unfolds.

iv. Skinny, Sexy EATING:

Splurge on a calorie indulgence that you love. Eat it in front of someone whom you would normally never eat dessert and taste how empowering it feels to eat without guilt and with full enjoyment. You might even find that the first few bites are so delightful that you don't need to finish your dessert.

v. Skinny, Sexy YOU:

Enjoying life takes confidence, but it also necessitates an innate openness to happiness. Decide that you deserve happiness, and be open to it. You must accept happiness in order to embrace the idea of self-confidence. Embrace this and you are on your way to living *skinny* and *sexy*.

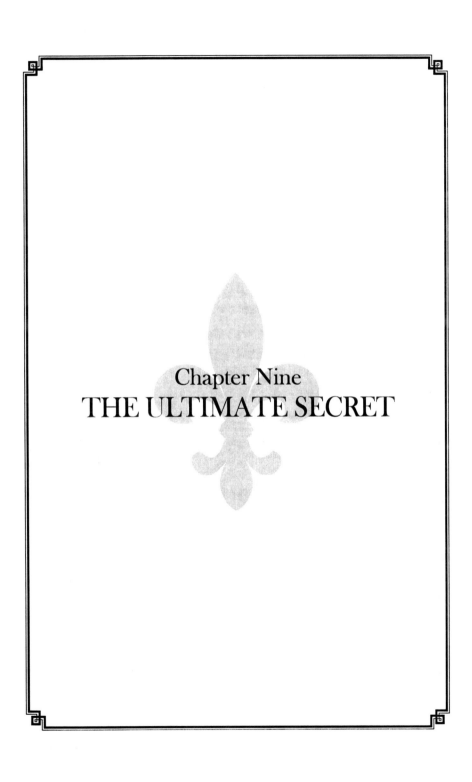

Chapter Nine
THE ULTIMATE SECRET

Chapter Nine
THE ULTIMATE SECRET

Now that we have defined the first element of *joie de vivre*, confidence, we must dissect the second essential element, balance, in
order to discover the ultimate French secret.

In understanding what true balance and body confidence are, we must
understand the powerful role they play in our lives and self-identity.
Appreciation for one's body comes only from a balanced view of the
body-mind-soul trinity of identity. Like anything that is misunderstood
or unappreciated, our bodies suffer when neglected or criticized.

We are beautiful, but we either do not believe in our beauty or we
are afraid of it. The cultural obsession with physical beauty has so
warped our understanding of ourselves that we trivialize the value
of our true natural beauty – that which is our true selves and lies in
our heart, personality and quirks.

America, the land of extremes, has lost its balance on beauty and
even the idea of balance at all. Physical and inner beauties are not
separate entities; rather, they flow out of one another and they are
part of one another.

When a woman has a firm understanding of her captivating inner
beauty, she finally is able to allow her soul to flow through her

skin, which gives her that mesmerizing physical glow that we all so desperately crave. She is that woman that is so alluring, confident, intriguing, and indisputably beautiful that men and women alike are fascinated. She is a gem.

There is silence about this imbalance in America. I see this silence in gyms, schools and in families. Our nation of girls and women is in desperate need of help. We are programming a nation to believe that our body defines our beauty. We teach our children that true beauty is on the inside, but we live as if true beauty only matters on the outside. By the time an American girl turns 12, she has been exposed to over 77,000 re-touched advertisements propagating media's standard of beauty. It is no wonder that by the age of 10, over 80% of girls admit to have a fear of becoming fat.

I want to share my client profile in order to further demonstrate this concept of balance. I am not singling out any particular client or gym, but rather a collective image of women I have met from Chicago, Illinois, Washington, D.C., and Charlotte, North Carolina. In general, I rarely come across a healthy, well-balanced woman with a healthy body, mind and spirit. I am not talking only about actual health, but also about personal body image. The two must go hand-in-hand. That being said, I do have healthy, balanced clients – unfortunately though, they are a minority.

An estimated 20% of those I meet with have a healthy mind and healthy body. If I were to categorize the other 80% of my clients, the word *balance* is unfortunately not one that would fit their description. These wonderful, struggling people fall into three distinct profiles healthy mind / unhealthy body, healthy body / unhealthy mind, and unhealthy body / unhealthy mind.

As the chapter title promises, we are going to define balance. Instead of a definition, I am going to start by giving you a definition of what balance is *not*.

The first category, healthy mind / unhealthy body is an interesting blend. This type of person has a strong sense of self, a distinctly loving family structure, and a firm grasp on the beauty of their individuality. Typically however, the state and health of their bodies fall low on their priority list. Healthy mind / unhealthy body people teeter-totter between being either extremely overweight or extremely underweight, never attaining their bodies' natural healthy weight of balance.

I will begin with the obvious healthy mind / unhealthy body example, those who are physically overweight. Three of the most entertaining and rambunctious clients I have ever trained were a group of three 30-something-year-old ladies. Athletic in their younger years, these ladies were full of life, confident in who they were, and made no excuses for the extra forty pounds of fat their bodies had grown accustomed to bearing. Confident and unabashedly excited about the gym, my ladies knighted themselves "Team Flab." With a healthier body weight as their goal, they were disciplined, hard workers and believed in laughing throughout the entirety of a workout. They trained with me for over three months and made great progress; they changed unhealthy eating and drinking habits, lost weight and descended in clothing sizes.

Then, one day they stopped coming. A week went by, a month went by, and a summer went by. Occasionally I would run into them at a restaurant: they would hang their heads in shame, and laugh about how crazy their schedules had become. It was true too, every one of the three worked in a management or regional directorship position, and all were involved in work-related travel on the weekends. But what is also true is that the gym was no longer a priority to them. Being healthy had, somehow, become a chore. The journey towards a lifestyle and body change that I had tried to instill in them fizzed out. "Change your body, change your life" no longer mattered to them as much as other things in their lives.

Are they well-adjusted, well-balanced, happy, beautiful women? Yes, extremely. Are their bodies as healthy as their minds? No. And that is their ticking time bomb.

Time cannot be an excuse in a lifestyle change. Time is the greatest currency we as human beings have ever been given. The beauty of currency is that it gives the individual the ability to *choose* where to spend it, and those choices simply fall into a hierarchy of needs, wants, obligations, and priorities.

The archenemy my Team Flab was my Team Skinny Fat. Skinny Fat, another healthy mind / unhealthy body, was comprised of two stunning, twenty-five year old women; one tall blond with long limbs, the other, petite brunette with pronounced dimples. The two teams dominated the gym social circles and joked appropriately about team rivalries.

The Skinny Fat girls were ladies with fun personalities and worked out with me at the gym in six-week stints between their trips to the Bahamas. Always tan, and always getting in better shape for their newest upgrade of Bahamian lover, they seemed untouchable.

The girls self-proclaimed themselves Skinny Fat after we discovered that their body fat analysis determined them to be borderline obese, even though the average passerby would deem them as skinny. Suddenly, when they discovered their dangerously high body fat percentages, the need to tone and build muscle wasn't simply for aesthetics, but for fundamental health reasons.

The whole skinny fat concept is where most young girls go wrong; in seeing someone who you deem to be skinny, you assume that they are healthy. Unfortunately, skinny people can be just as unhealthy as the obese. Their arteries are just as easily blocked by built-up cholesterol, they are equally prone to cardiovascular disease, and are equivalently lethargic and out of shape. We need to redefine our understanding of "skinny" and instead pursue healthy bodies, and *skinny, sexy minds.*

Team Skinny Fat began to get toned; they made small changes in their daily lives and they were pleased with their new commitment to health. Then, life hit. Time took over, and they stopped coming to the gym. Their flattened tummies filled out and their tightening legs got a bit looser. I haven't seen them since.

People tend to be jealous of the naturally skinny, and they don't let that go unknown. It is too easy for an unhealthy skinny person to stop exercising and stop eating healthy, because, well, it is almost socially acceptable and because they can get away with it if appearance is the goal.

Whether someone is skinny, overweight, or somewhere in between, doesn't prove that they have a healthy or unhealthy body image. It is quite the contrary actually. The number of women who struggle with some facet of an eating disorder is rising drastically in the United States with each year that passes. The National Association of Anorexia Nervosa and Associated Disorders (ANAD) recently released statistics in which they estimate that there are currently 24 million Americans suffering from anorexia, bulimia and binge eating disorder. Add that to the millions of American women and men with an Eating Disorder Not Otherwise Specified (EDNOS), and you realize how many millions of Americans are walking around hating the skin they are in.

These women and men, caught in a constant battlefield of the mind, struggle tremendously with food. They fight with themselves over food, exercise, and every daily activity, clutching desperately to find contentment with their bodies. These are the women that can be labeled into the healthy body / unhealthy mind group. The healthy body / unhealthy mind group can include any shape, size or color, and those who could be classified as healthy body / unhealthy minds are oftentimes adept at on putting on a façade of confidence.

Women who are healthy body / unhealthy minds are muddied up in a body-esteem crisis. They are physically fit and externally beautiful, but have absolutely no true confidence or inner sense of self. In a nutshell, these women fall prey to their greatest fears of rejection, abandonment, and just not measuring up.

We are so desperately afraid of not being loved or accepted for our true selves that our healthy body / unhealthy minds hone in on our physical imperfections as a scapegoat form of protection. Subconsciously, we prescribe to the mindset that a perfect body will guarantee us love, commitment, and freedom from our innate fear of rejection. In the case that we are discarded by someone we love, we are able to convince ourselves that it never has to do with our true identity; it is simply because our bodies are a disappointment. It is our minds' own little intuitive way of protecting our souls' vulnerability. Unfortunately, instead of protecting ourselves, we end up destroying our spirits and hating our bodies.

I am one such healthy body / unhealthy mind women. So is one of my dear high school friends, whom I will call Belle. Belle was an elite athlete, brilliant student, and beautiful. She came from a distinguished family and her college years were spent being academically and athletically successful at one of the top liberal arts schools in the nation. Belle and I went to different colleges, however, when I visited her on weekends I learned that she still lived in the same destructive habits of obsession as her high school days. She trained for her sport about four hours a day and made a habit of running an extra hour on her own at night instead of going to the fraternity houses with her friends.

Belle was an obsessive calorie counter and exercised just as compulsively. The most unique thing about Belle was that she rarely ate normal portion sizes when around others. At meals she would make a small plate and then pick from everyone else's. Nighttime for Belle, as for me, was her nemesis. When dusk fell, so did Belle's guard. Binges were easy to hide and early morning runs on the treadmill could negate the guilt that plagued her. So self-critical, Belle preferred to stay to herself and while clearly very socially involved, was never very social per se. Belle would never admit that she has disordered eating. Belle was the perfect pretender.

Another example of a health body / unhealthy mind close to my heart is a 20-year-old brunette named Jordan. I see her at the gym every day; she is at the center of the circle of testosterone pumped college boys who are desperate in their efforts to win her attention. Jordan is a ditzy sweetheart and knows every staff member in the gym. Jordan didn't stick out to me, though, because I thought she was nice, but because she reminded me of myself and that scared me.

Jordan is at the gym almost more than I am, and I work sixty-hour weeks. I have seen her there seven days a week, usually twice a day, and always doing the same three cardio machines: the seated bike, the Precor elliptical, and another seated bike in a different location. It never fails, and her body never changes.

Jordan almost became a client of mine, but was too scared to change her routine as she knew I would ask her to do, so she continues with her cardio obsession. She is afraid of lifting weights, and afraid to eat more than two times a day. Determined to lose 20 pounds and 7% body fat (she wants that toned look you see in magazines, she told me), she is terrified to stop her daily three hours of cardio.

Even after an explanation of how to properly train the body – with weights, cardio, proper nutrition, and proper rest – she continues paralyzed in her routine. Jordan confesses she feels imprisoned. Her legs disgust her; her self-hatred has warped her entire perception of self. She is even unreceptive and unaware of the number of young men who drool over what they consider to be her perfection.

Her greatest struggle is her fear to eat. She never eats more than 1,000 calories a day. Jordan admits that she needs to stop watch-ing MTV, and her favorite show, *The Hills*, but doesn't have the willpower to do so and is equally fearful of falling out of the loop socially with friends who are equally hooked to MTV culture. Jordan has a long sentence ahead of her and will only find freedom when her desperation meets the courage and maturity required to change. Unfortunately, Jordan is far from freedom because she, like many healthy body / unhealthy minds, lives in denial.

Most healthy body / unhealthy minds that I know personally live in denial with what I consider to be their own mental prison. They endure this entrapment for years before acknowledging to themselves that they want to change. Jordan estimated that over 90% of her daily thought life is spent on thinking about calories, her next meal, or her next workout. Disordered eating and body image not only consume the body, but they steal life.

Jordan knows she needs to change. But there is a distinct difference between *needing* to change and *wanting* to change. She knows that her current lifestyle is a secret addiction, an addiction to exercise and to self-loathing, and that it is making her miserable. Fear, however, makes Jordan afraid to take the first true step of change, which is the step of acknowledgement. Jordan must decide that she wants to change – truly change at the depth of her core.

Finally, we come to the category of unhealthy mind / unhealthy body, the group I love to love on the most. These are the women and men who are desolate; it is a group of beautiful people that America has given up on and judges very harshly. Just a brief look into the eyes of an unhealthy mind / unhealthy body reveals hidden pains of their past and deeply pervasive emotional scars. What is interesting about unhealthy mind / unhealthy body scars is that, no matter where they originate from, they blemish both mind and body and distort the person's entire understanding of themselves and their role as a loved human being. My unhealthy mind / unhealthy body clients have endured lifetimes of callous name-calling, years of verbal abuse, disparagement from loved ones, and discouraging statement from doctors, insurance companies and even airlines. Unhealthy mind / unhealthy bodies are so accustomed to being criticized, labeled, and judged by society that they ultimately see themselves as what other people see physically. Many admit to me that they feel invisible to the world.

Most people who meet Francie, one of my unhealthy mind / unhealthy body clients, would describe her as "sunny." Petit and plump, she wears joy through her smile and is welcoming and witty with every stranger she meets. When she comes to the gym to see me, she bellows *"Hi Sunshine!!!"* out to me from across the entire facility.

Francie has been overweight her entire life, ever since a traumatic life-defining event happened to her as a young child. Since that pinpointed moment in time, Francie, Little Miss Sunshine herself, has retreated to eating as a form of self-protection and self-preservation. As a child, she was heavily criticized for her weight by someone abusively controlling in her life. While this person belittled her worth, she found safety in food. Her morphing and growing body kept her safe from harm's way, and gave her a physical reason to hate herself.

Well-adjusted and generally confident, Francie has lived life well as a large woman. But, Francie is a pretender. Some days she knows that she is beautiful, in fact, if you did not know her, you would say that she is sassy and confident like a Hollywood starlet. Other days, Francie sees herself as a terrified little girl warily hiding from the world behind a layer of fat. Those are the days when she loses who she is, when she forgets that what really defines her beauty is on the inside. She knows she is beautiful though in fact some days she is sassy and more confident than some Hollywood stars. Other days, Francie sees herself as a terrified little girl warily hiding from the world behind a layer of fat. Those are the days when she loses who she is, when she forgets that what defines her is simply that: *her*, not how much she currently weighs.

Recently, Francie had her stomach banded, a less invasive procedure than gastric bypass. Much weight loss ensued, but to reach her healthy body weight, Francie has 100 more pounds to lose. She sweats her heart and soul out at the gym and has committed herself to a total life change.

The journey to health for Francie has numerous obstacles and there will undoubtedly have countless to come, because, you see, Francie is still fighting to mentally and emotionally break free from identifying herself with her actual skin.

Speaking of skin, we must stop confining ourselves to ours. We are so much deeper and more wonderful than the circumference, elasticity and clarity of our skin; we all know that fundamentally, but why can't we live it and truly believe it?

A few extra inches of skin have mentally plagued another one of my unhealthy mind / unhealthy body clients. Lulu is no ordinary weight-loss client; Lulu lost 100 pounds on her own by simple dietary changes *before* she even came to see me. Lulu lost 50 additional pounds after a few months of spending six days a week with me at the gym. She has achieved no ordinary feat and she looks like a completely different person today than she did two years ago. Although she made such drastic changes for her own personal health, she did it also out of love for her husband and two little girls. It was not a change based on vanity for Lulu – no, Lulu is too intellectual and too deep to be bothered by such trivialities.

However, what has haunted Lulu is an inch of excess skin that hangs from her triceps, which, after such dramatic weight loss and body composition change, is only to be expected. In such a scenario, typically, the most efficient way to redevelop elasticity and to tighten the skin is by actually removing the excess through surgery. Lulu understands that, but does not want anything to do with surgery, for that would be too vain.

The trouble is that Lulu still sees herself as a 300-pound women and she hides her arms in shame. It is not until that shame of her past disappears that Lulu will finally see herself for who she is and who she has always been. The choice is hers, just as we each have a choice. We will either hold on to our insecurities, allowing them to steal away our life and joy, or accept them and start seeing ourselves and the world with new, fresh, *kind* eyes. Again, it is our choice that determines our destiny.

French women take great pride in those little things that bring a secret smile to oneself – the little pleasures that no one but you know about.

It is time that we each unleash our inner French hedonism; start small and start savoring. In order to best understand how start releasing your own inner hedonist, it is important to learn what category of mind-body relationship you fit. Please use the quiz below to determine where you fall and what aspect you need to most focus on in order to embrace your full *joie de vivre*.

THE HEALTHY MIND – HEALTHY BODY QUIZ

<u>How to take the quiz</u>: *Score 3 points per Mind / Body category to determine your current healthy mind – healthy body state.*

Possible Categories: (1) Healthy mind (2) Unhealthy mind (3) Healthy body (4) Unhealthy body

- Are you overweight or underweight?
  [Yes = 1 point (Category 4) / No= 1 point (Category 3)]

- Have you tried more than three diets in the past five years?
  [Yes =1 point (Category 4) / No = 1 point (Category 3)]

- Do you intentionally skip breakfast or any other meals?
  [Yes = 1 point (Category 4) / No= 1 point (Category 3)]

- Have you maintained your current weight for over six months and feel comfortable at your current size?
  [Yes= 1 point (Category 3)/ No= 1 point (Category 4)]

- Do you exercise consistently (and not obsessively strictly for calorie burn)?
  [Yes = 1 point (Category 3) / No = 1 point (Category 4)]

- Do you have disordered eating patterns or an eating disorder?
  [Yes = 1 point (Category 2) / No = 1 point (Category 1)]

- Do you weigh yourself more than once per week?
  [Yes = 1 point (Category 2)/ No = 1 point (Category 1)]

- Do you pay attention to the nutrient value of what you eat?
  [Yes = 1 point (Category 1) / No = 1 point (Category 2)]

- Do you eat whatever is available and easiest?
  [Yes = 1 point (Category 2) / No = 1 point (Category 1)]

- Do you get nervous thinking about getting in a bathing suit?
  [Yes = 1 point (Category 2) /No = 1 point (Category 1)]

An article in the July 2008 edition of *Glamour* (France edition) divulged the insecurities that French women struggle with. Each woman interviewed explained her complex, how it had mentally plagued her in her past, and summarized how she overcame her body-complex.

The verb *s'assumer* was each woman's word of choice concerning her self-acceptance and triumph. *S'assumer,* literally "to come to terms with oneself," carries a depth of self-acceptance that the English language cannot summarize so simplistically. The phrase *"je m'assume,"* or *"je l'assume,"* translates into the idea that one takes responsibility for oneself, or has come to terms with something.

Counter to the women's confessions, *Glamour* revealed the results of a survey taken among French men concerning their views of women's bodies and unique characteristics. Seventy percentage of Frenchmen expressed that they found perfection in the bodies of women that they interacted with on a daily basis, and found that women who obsessed over weight to be *"ennuyeuese,"* or annoying. In France, women strive to *bein dans leur peau* and avoid being categorized as *ennuyeuse,* but is important to note that even the French have to make a daily, conscientious effort to love the skin they are in. André Manoukian, a production specialist, commented about women's bodies:

> They have internalized a social regard and critique of beauty now shared from Shanghai to New York, among the rich and among the poor. Their unique, perfect body has just contradicted ours. Women no longer persecute themselves in the name of God, but rather in accordance to a new way: the religion of esthetics. With individualism, we live in the self-construction of one's own image. One is responsible for one's self, therefore of one's body, and thus, one's weight… from where comes an anxiety without limits. Me, I like curves because the charm of the body, that is to be excessive. Skinniness corresponds with the great modern fantasy: speed, lightness, escape from the material; the paradox being anorexia. In short, the style returns despite its platonic rhetoric: the souls are imprisoned inside the body. *(author's translation)*

He brilliantly summarizes the simple truth that men find us more attractive in our uniqueness, and not in spite of our blemishes but because of them. He parallels the curves of a woman's body to an invitation to become enveloped within that curvaceous body. Another man, Pascal Bruckner, lamented that "women judge themselves with cruelty." He intuitively assessed:

> It's a shame, because men are more attached to the characteristics [of a woman] that are a bit off. A leg, an arm, a shoulder, that expresses something that proves it is flesh. Consider a breast that juts out: one wants only to confide in it! *(author's translation)*

Clearly, as Bruckner's confessions reveal, French women are not exempt from the self-imposed judgment and cruelty we American women bring upon ourselves. However, some take charge of their beauty in a different way than we do in America. French women are starting to get caught in the social epidemic of streamlined beauty that flows in media images from Shanghai to New York.

Bruckner coins this phenomenon as the "religion of esthetics." This is a twisted sense of individualism; the desire of ownership and self-construction. Be aware of the idea of individual strength and beauty is tainted by our subscription to a dangerous standard of unnatural, photo-shopped beauty.

According to Frenchwoman Hortense de Monplaisir, a woman has the ability to take charge of her beauty, and to self-construct in a healthier, yet still individualistic manner. She suggests doing so via simple pleasures. She confesses in her comical book *Le Dossier, How to Survive the English*:

> I would say that no woman can afford to pass up the op-portunity to feel *éclatante et seduisante*; and when in Paris, I always buy a little something at Fifi Chohnil on the rue St-Honoré

So rather than hound herself on her imperfections, she suggests acceptance and indulgence. Actually, she implies that every woman needs to feel "brilliant" and "seductive" to feel fully feminine and fully alive. In other words, accept yourself and identify the small things that bring you pleasure. Many of us are so busy that we have forgotten how to feel brilliant about ourselves.

The ultimate French secret is their uncanny ability to love, and to be comfortable in the skin they are in.

Incorporate the following suggestions and you will start to rediscover your own brilliance.

DISCOVERING YOUR OWN BRILLANCE:

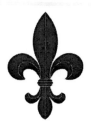

- Spoil yourself in small things that bring you great pleasure.

- Invest in quality.

- Lavish your tummy and thighs; caress them each morning and evening with the finest cream you own. You will start to see those parts more kindly, and you will even start to like them.

- Invest in matching lingerie. You will be pleasantly surprised in the restroom on a Monday morning when you're feeling frumpy but find yourself secretly smiling at your sexy ensemble that only you know about.

- Indulge in those things that make you feel stunning and seductive; own your beauty from the smallest details and have your beauty be for yourself.

- Never shave your legs for a man; shave your legs because the smoothness makes you feel like a woman.

French hedonism and the idea of pleasure play an essential role in the development and balance of a Frenchwoman's self-perception. Hedonism in moderation, the ultimate pursuit of pleasure, can be a positive way to love your life and have a healthy affect on others.

Remember, the ultimate French secret is found in knowing how to live comfortably in your own skin. This secret is one that must be discovered through first-hand experiences and cannot just be told. My discovery of this secret resulted from my combined experiences in France. One of my very first lessons in the unveiling of the secret came in the form of a wine lesson.

Natalie, Christine, Clémence, and Sébastian, my French co-workers, each shared their own love of gastronomy and oenology with me. In every course and glass of wine that was shared, I received a compilation of lessons in the process of learning to slow down, taste and appreciate what was truly being shared. They teased me for being the overly eager American in my efforts to understand wine tasting. Instead, they urged me to be patient, to engage my senses, and to learn the distinctions myself through my own tastes, smells, memories and senses. Rather than having a textbook knowledge of their wine and their lives, they wanted me to develop my own understanding and my own interpretation. Leave it to the French to demand that I am an individual; they wanted my opinion on things, not simply a repeated opinion from someone else.

They were the example I emulated as I embraced each delightful piece of French tradition in my tastings. Yes, appreciation can be learned; however, you must be willing to learn slowly, as I did. I spent many evenings trying to keep up in conversations that jumped from Saint Emilion vintages to lycée politics to the most recent literary release, desperately trying to remain engaged and to contribute my own thoughts to the discussion.

Inevitably, mid-debate, they would then turn to me and ask what I thought of the Guyère combined with the 1997 Bourgogne, I would grapple to recall as many details as I could without confusing it with the four other vintages I had drank. In order to keep up and formulate my own taste memories and opinions, I had to slow down and savor. As you learn slowly to appreciate textures and tastes, you will in turn learn to appreciate and discover yourself in a similar manner.

As I did, we can all learn from the example the French have given us in their love for sharing and discovering wine. There are five basic steps in tasting wine: seeing, swirling, sniffing, sipping, and savoring. In the journey of self-discovery and body acceptance, these steps can parallel the unveiling of ourselves as well.

When we *see* ourselves, we need to ask what we see. Do we see through the mirror, with our own eyes, with the eyes of others, or with our hearts? Some of us never advance past this step of seeing, so caught up are we in external appearances and perceptions that we lose our ability to progress. This is the great danger so many woman struggle with today: judging ourselves based on socially set standards. Our external self-judgment stunts our ability to develop, or, in keeping with the wine analogy, age. Everyone knows the more aged the wine is, the better is tastes. For the human, the more aged (and self-aware) the individual, the more they have the ability to truly taste and enjoy what life has to give.

Start seeing yourself with kind eyes, for it is only once you do that you will be able to swirl what you see, and enjoy the complexity of the swirl.

Now, it is time to *swirl* our identities: that is, to consider whether or not we are who we are because of what others tell us or because of we really know ourselves. We all are raised with some inherited concept of our identities, or at least of what our families wish us to be. Challenge your past conceptions of yourself, challenge your placement in social circles, and really challenge yourself to swirl around ideas of what exactly makes you *you*.

Sniffing involves understanding yourself on a multiple level of senses and it is the development of extended self-awareness – becoming three dimensional to oneself. Familiarizing yourself with the aromas associated with the characteristics of humanity, you will learn to appreciate your senses to the fullest.

Breathe in deeply and count to seven; exhale deeply. What does it feel like to fully inflate your lunges? Do it and take a moment to analyze how you it makes you feel. This is the process in which we become familiar with ourselves. Get familiar with yourself. Settle in to your senses and start trying to identify the verbiage that describes each and every sensation you feel. If it makes you feel alive, describe that. It makes me feel alive; I feel my ribs, I am aware of my bone structure, and I feel my body interacting as a fusion, a miracle. I exhale greatness. I exhale life. What do you exhale?

As you progress through the wine tasting process of discovery, you will come to the stage of actually *sipping*. When you sip, you bring life and vibrancy to your lips. This is the stage of experimentation, the stage of discovery. Sipping is the art of appreciation; there is no greed, there is no deadline, and there is no judgment. It is OK to reject something, to disagree with it, or to define your own preferences. What is important is that you explore your world of senses and experiences and that you are not afraid to expand your understanding of the world around you. In better understanding the diversity of the world around you, you will also better understand yourself.

Finally, we arrive at the moment to which all other four stages build up to – the ability to appreciate the wine. Like the way in which you savor the final taste of the wine rising upon the roof of your mouth, so too *savor* life. Allow the emotions, wounds, joys, and circumstances in your life that shape you to swish around in your mouth enough that you find the exquisite artistry in their combination. You will begin to see the beautiful chaos that makes your life so unique and you will begin to see your body as a reflection of the years of experience and life you have lived.

The only thing holding you back in life is you. Discover yourself. Live yourself. Savor yourself. Experience yourself and then express what you feel to others. Be proud of who you are and of what you are interested in. You are unstoppable, because, if you have followed this guideline of tasting, you are in the process of tasting life.

Nothing more, nothing less, just tasting life; so stop over-analyzing everything you do and everyone around you, stop burdening yourself with negative fears, and just taste.

THE ULTIMATE FRENCH SECRET
Skinny, Sexy à la carte
Le soleil luit pour tout le monde.
[The sun shines for one and all.]

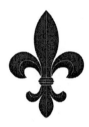

i. Skinny, Sexy SUMMARY:

The ultimate secret to French confidence is living comfortably and confidently in one's own skin. America, the land of extremes, has lost its balance on beauty and even the idea of balance at all. The French have a concept of personal balance and acceptance engrained into their culture, literally they "come to terms" with themselves, or, in other words, they *s'assumer. S'assume*r, literally "to come to terms with oneself," carries a depth of self-acceptance that the English language cannot summarize so sophistically.

ii. Skinny, Sexy REFLECTION:

Do you accept yourself for who you are, in all your quirks, physical traits and perfect imperfections? *If not, what is holding you back?* What would it take for you to let go of obsessing over perfection and to start seeing yourself as a balanced whole?

iii. Skinny, Sexy PERSONAL APPLICATION:

It's time to take charge of your own beauty and brilliance. Commit to trying all six suggestions provided in the insert of this chapter to work towards discovering what it is that makes being you so great.

iv. Skinny, Sexy EATING:

Strive for a healthy mind and healthy body. If you think that you have disordered eating tendencies, tell someone and seek professional help.

v. Skinny, Sexy YOU:

French hedonism, the ultimate balanced pursuit of pleasure, can be a positive way to love your life. As you love your life and yourself, your confidence will soar and you will start having a healthy affect on others.

Try to find new ways to be comfortable in the skin you are in. Be creative: try new styles of clothes, new thought patterns, new foods. The only thing holding you back in life is you. Discover yourself. Love yourself. Love the skin you are in. It starts for you today if you decide that you want it to.

Chapter Ten
YOUR JOURNEY OF BEAUTY
AND BODY SHAPE

Chapter Ten
YOUR JOURNEY OF BEAUTY
AND BODY SHAPE

Most of us are aware that beauty is in the eye of the beholder. The question is do we allow others to be our beholders? Also, are we responsible and self-aware enough to embrace and define our own beauty? In other words, are you your own beholder?

Remember, the ultimate French secret is that life is meant to be lived *comfortably* and *confidently* in your own skin. That means embracing your skin and the fluctuations of your body shape without allowing any smidgen of self-consciousness to interfere with your ability to live life to the fullest.

Living life, like many other things, is a choice. Living is an action, a verb, and therefore, an active choice that we make daily. Any form of self-consciousness, fear or body image preoccupation will quickly impede your ability live out loud. It throws us into a sort of mental paralysis that impedes our ability to live. For many, the instant a self-doubting thought enters our mind; we transition to "autopilot." We simply go into survival mode and try to just make it through the day.

Autopilot is not a verb; it is a noun. Autopilot is not living. Life is meant to be a verb, and the French know that. It is time that we, too, catch on.

Any time I have ever doubted myself or been distracted by self-consciousness, I have wasted a full day. I have allowed myself to transition into autopilot mode and I chose, for that day, not to fully live. When we are in autopilot, we focus on the negative rather than the positive. Many of us will think about the pudge in our tummy so much that it steals our entire confidence. Our own negative thoughts steal the strength away from our identity. It is human nature that autopilot runs with a predisposition to negativity. Turn off this survival mechanism and realize that life isn't meant to be survived. It is meant to be lived.

How many days of your life have you been on autopilot? Moreover, in any given week, how many days do you *live* and how many days do you autopilot yourself?

These are hard questions to grasp. Be honest with yourself and realize that you are on the narrow path to true living. The promenade to *joie de vivre* is very different than what you may be used to, so it will feel funny at first. Embrace it and keep following your heart; you will not regret it.

Learning to be your own beholder begins with looking in the mirror and accepting who you are and the things you cannot change. In accepting the things about yourself that you cannot change, you will discover a newfound peace. With peace comes freedom, and with freedom comes our ability to choose. The power of choice gives you the strength and ability to choose *life* every day.

I am 5'4" and used to wish that I was 5'9." I have never loved being short. I have muscular legs; they are powerhouses that have given me much success athletically. I went through a phase in college where I berated myself for not "having the body" or height to be able to wear Capris, skinny jeans, or short skirts like some of my friends. The moment, years later, when I finally accepted that my legs were *meant* to be short and that there is nothing I can possibly do to ever change them, I experienced a breakthrough in confidence. I learned to love what clothes and cuts did flatter my petit frame and actually arrived at a point of thankfulness for my five foot four stance. In fact, I am now proud of my toned legs and find incredible beauty in their shape, strength and flexibility. I like being petite in build and I simply have accepted that Capris were not designed for my body.

Is there something about your body that you are holding against yourself? Imagine what life will be like when you are able to accept that as a unique part of your beauty. Self-acceptance is a lot easier said than done, but it must begin somewhere.

The second step in body-acceptance is to find every beautiful thing there is about your body and write it down. Write it down and say it out loud. As I have recommended before, make a list. You will be amazed at how this list will come to be useful on days when you are just not feeling like yourself or on days that you are a little bit down and out. Take time thinking about your body and come up with twenty different things about you physically that make you beautifully and undeniably you!

TWENTY THINGS I LOVE ABOUT MY BODY:

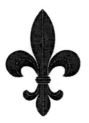

1. _____

2. _____

3. _____

4. _____

5. _____

6. _____

7. _____

8. _____

9. _____

10. _____

11. _____

12. _____

13. _____

14. _____

15. _____

16. _____

17. _____

18. _____

19. _____

20. _____

When you find self-negativity and old thought-patterns encroaching, it is time to realign your Zen. A concept from Chinese Buddhism, Zen is enlightenment by meditation where there is no consciousness of self. Imagine how free, alive, and fulfilled you can feel in your skin if you are able to reach a point where your subconscious allows your mind to achieve peace and balance.

To realign your Zen, allow your brain to edit and cleanse negativity by doing anything that makes you feel at peace. Zen can come in a lavender bath, a car ride with the windows down, a run with your favorite music pumping, prayer, a cup of tea, with a hug or through uplifting conversation with a friend. Whatever it is that brings you to that point of peace, do it. Peace will cleanse your thoughts and self-criticisms and will sharpen your eye for beauty in both yourself and the world around you.

Be your own beholder of beauty; doing so will free you to live comfortably and healthily in your own skin.

YOU AND THE THREE TYPES OF BEAUTY

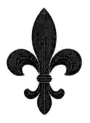

A wise friend once told me that "pretty" is boring. She is right, but many of us live unaware of the distinction between pretty and beautiful. We spend hours of our day striving to be pretty, to look like our peers and to fit in, and meanwhile we don't realize how boring such homogeneity really is. Instead, I encourage you to seek out beauty, the beauty that makes you dynamically you and definitely not boring. You must take ownership of your inner beauty for it to reflect outward.

I have come to believe that there are three types of beauty: external beauty, internal beauty, and life beauty. The truly beautiful woman has the full trinity of this beauty, each inter-dependent upon the other types. External beauty is magnified by inner beauty and life beauty can only be appreciated through the lens of confident inner beauty. Finally, external beauty contributes to life beauty. The same wise friend describes beauty as beauty in action. Beauty is not necessarily something you can capture in a still photograph; rather, it is something in motion, in movement and fully alive.

The power of a positive word of affirmation cannot be underestimated. For some, it could be a difference between life and death. Knowing that you are not the only one to struggle with personal conflicts of beauty, body acceptance, and purpose should give you a sense of hope and solidarity. Share that hope by affirming and loving those around you, even strangers.

I am convinced that as women we are so preoccupied with our external beauty that we are unaware of the other two types of beauty needed to make us feel complete. How many women do you know, when asked how things are going, would reply: "life is beautiful." Most people that I know tend to be exasperated, over-worked, over-scheduled, and stressed out. Sure, people have good vacations, or nice weekends, or a good day every now and then, but how many people do you know genuinely emanate a joy of living?

When you meet someone who loves life, you will know it. It shines through them, through their eyes, and through their smile. It is as if their heart is more sensitive to others and they have a polarized ability to attract others to them.

Be one of those people. How, you ask? It starts with ownership of self. Take pride in who you are and in what makes you tick. Own your beauty. Define what beauty is to you, and remember that what it is to you might be different from what it is to someone else. Be confident in what brings pleasure to your eyes and seek to discover the way in which the beauty and uniqueness of your personality speaks through your style, your smile, and even your scent.

Also, relish in your "flaws," they are what make you more approachable and real to others. By embracing your insecurities, you will claim ownership over them. In doing so, your flaw will have no self-sabotaging power over you, and, conversely, it will become one of your characteristic strengths. Your confidence in your inner beauty will begin to magnify your external beauty, and your eyes will finally open to seeing life itself from a fresh perspective of beauty.

Beauty is an inter-dependent cycle that depends upon your personal decision to love yourself for who you are. The rivers of beauty and *joie de vivre* will begin to flow from that moment on. It is a beautiful experience and will not go unnoticed by those in your life.

When I think about this cyclical beauty, I think of my French co-worker Clémence. Clémence was quirky and enthusiastic, the perfect type of teacher for a first grade class. Petite with wild curly hair and typically dressed in five layers of bohemian scarves, Clémence had style. I interacted with her both inside and outside work, and her demeanor never changed. She was always bubbly, always smiling, and always comfortable in her skin. The more I learned about Clémence, the more I respected her *joie*. It turns out that when I came into Clémence's life, she was in the middle of a nasty separation with her fiancée and was under some heavy financial burdens as well. You would have never known her circumstances, for Clémence's inner beauty was so defined that she didn't waver at the external changes that she was confronting in her daily environment. Clémence was happy to just be, and her *joie* was contagious.

Remember, beauty should not be definable by societal standards. Beauty is defined subjectively and with each individual. It is in the eye of the beholder. Be your own beholder. When you focus all your energy on changing the beauty you already possess and in hating your current body, you are wishing your existence and your uniqueness away. When you wish away what you were blessed with, you negate the power of your natural beauty. This is probably the greatest distinction between American and French women. We get sucked into the cycle of homogenizing our bodies and beauty while the French accept the skin they're in, allowing their spirits and natural beauty to emanate. Women who only strive for physical perfection end up wasting the goodness and grace others already see in them.

DISCOVERING YOUR BEAUTY TYPE

So, I ask, in terms of beauty, what is your priority in life? Which of the three types of beauty do you think about most? In dwelling on this (and yes, please dwell – remember the European mentality and proceed slowly and naturally), let these following questions cascade through your thoughts to help in this stage of self-reflection:

What is the difference between your stated priorities and true priorities in life? What would an outsider say when observing you?

Remember, the only way to have a *skinny, sexy mind* is to have another purpose in life. How have you chosen your purpose in life? Are you a person of consistency? Is your life purpose the same in the morning when you first rise, mid-afternoon in the bustle of your day, and in evening as you relax? A person of consistency is a peaceful person.

I have to make a conscious decision on a daily basis to choose to love my body. I choose to be at peace with my body and to allow my natural beauty to shine through my smile. I do it by dwelling on the *joie* I find in being alive, being able to move, and being distinctly beautiful in my own way.

Ask yourself what it is that makes you relax, that takes down your defensive fronts, that relieves anxiety, that brings you contentment: that, my friend, needs to be a priority in your life. It could be watching a movie with your family, going for a run, taking a bath, reading, sharing a glass of wine with your loved one, or writing. Again, it is simply finding your Zen.

Finding what relaxation means to you is your first clue in understanding your purpose for existing. Relaxation will enable you to become more attuned to your body's needs and will enable you to build a deeper sense of appreciation for your body shape as you realize how wonderfully your body serves you. There is an incredible tie between body acceptance, body confidence and sense of purpose that many are unaware of. Most people, men and women included, struggle with this type of confidence. Truthfully, it is more an issue of lost purpose than of confidence. A person with a purpose is a person that will naturally be filled with confidence for the simple reason that he or she has a purpose in living. What do you do in your alone time?

Alone time is precious and what we do with it often demonstrates how we see ourselves. What we do in our leisure is among what we value most in our identity. Remember, time is the most valuable currency in the world; it is something that once spent, can never be gotten back. Is your alone time usually positive or negative? Many body image sufferers struggle when they are alone. If you are binging, over-eating, or numbing yourself into an alcoholic stupor, then you are running away from your true self. You are running from you anxieties by using food or substance as a drug. Drugs impede life.

Our ultimate goal of true happiness and body confidence is found in the ability to simply live for the sake of enjoying life. Permit me to use my past as an example: being a young single twenty-something, nights when I was home alone were an emotional coin toss. Some nights I was very inspired to write, to take a long, luxurious bath, or to catch up with old friends on the phone over a glass of wine. Other nights I struggled. It was a slippery mood to identify: a combination of fear, loneliness, anxiety and sabotage, my inner coward emerged.

Everyone's cowardly lion is unique. Mine attacks me when I am feeling unproductive, unattractive, and un-influential. It attacks my body shape and body value. I am besieged by self-doubt on the days when I question whether or not I have something great enough to share as a writer. The moments when I would long for a relationship, wish I was being more social or influential, or the times when I have any other sort of self-doubt, I yearned to numb myself. Numbness is an outlet; a way to escape the pain of uncertainty, awkwardness and doubt. Like any drug or addiction, numbness only makes me want to become more numb.

Ultimately we all struggle with a desire for a greater purpose. I yearn for purpose. We all yearn for purpose. I want to understand my identity and my meaning. The times when I don't are the times when I give up on myself and on my individuality. It is those times that I prescribe to the media-imposed standard bestowed upon me by society, and my body-confidence plummets. Living life without passion and purpose is like not existing. It is within our power to choose to exist and to choose to explore our purpose. You have the power to make things happen in your life, you just have to make the decision to believe in yourself in order to do it.

Be proactive. Be you! Your life is a blank page and you hold the pen. Write confidence for yourself, write joy, and write purpose.

BODY SHAPE AND
BODY BUMMING

In life, there is a way to live that is living, and a way to live that is just life. Each person chooses the path they wish to follow and every person prescribes to a certain lifestyle of priorities and focuses.

Beauty is and always has been worshipped by humankind. Yes, beauty is in the eye of the beholder, but what I am asserting here is that every beholder is continually seeking beauty. It is part of our nature, part of what drives us as human beings. It is undeniable that beauty ranks high in our understanding of life's purposes and priorities.

We pursue beauty in our surroundings and seek it out in our partners and friends. We nourish the development of inner beauty in the souls of our children, and continually seek to improve our own standard of physical attraction. We seek exotic vacation destinations in the Caribbean, dream of picnicking in the Swiss Alps, and long to travel the grainy dunes of the Sahara on camelback. We were programmed to yearn for that which is beautiful. The pursuit of beauty is part of what fills us with *joie de vivre*.

So even though we as Americans don't realize it, we too can master the French *joie de vivre* because it is naturally ingrained in us. Perhaps it would be better called *beauté de vivre*, because that is what we are all capable, if made aware. We are all capable of experiencing the *beauty* of living. The French word *vivre* is the infinite verb form, practically calling us to action. Within the phrases of *joie de vivre, beauté de vivre* and *rhythm de vivre*, there are outstanding implications of a demand to action, a call to life and a command to active living.

Beauty, though, when misunderstood, can be abused and neglected. More than that, it can be abusive. I am speaking here of un-owned beauty. Un-owned beauty is the beauty that exists within a person that the person is either not aware of or too critical of that causes them to ultimately reject themselves entirely.

> When beauty, our true light and power beyond measure, is un-owned, it is tragic.

I am witness to this type of beauty all too frequently. It shines through a woman when she cowers from her reflection in the mirror. It is evident in the over-coiffed, couture-dressed woman that refuses to step into public without layering on make-up. It yells out from the darkness of the bathroom from the thousands of bulimic women who fear and throw up the food they eat. Even the most well balanced women are subject to this plague: they are those who see themselves as simply "average."Embracing being average is like disowning yourself and your uniqueness. To be honest, battling "averageness" is no different from the battle of someone who struggles with an eating disorder. They are both ultimately the same – a rejection of your incredibly unique and beautiful self. When you think you are just average you are betraying the essence of your identity and ultimately your potential to truly impact the world.

Body bumming, the feeling of being bummed out about how you feel in your skin at any given time, occurs as a result of measuring your individual self-worth based upon a physical appearance or on societal praise.

I want to share with you the stories of two different, yet very similar women whom I was honored to befriend during my time in the fitness industry.

The first, whom I will call Rebecca, was one of the most beautiful women I have ever seen. She had beach-tanned skin, perfect dimensions, long legs, a chiseled stomach, and a gorgeous smile. Happily married to a well-established man, she owned her own business and could have easily been mistaken for a fitness model. She was so physically beautiful that it was intimidating. That was the Rebecca on the outside.

The real Rebecca was tragically trapped by her quest for perfection. Addicted to fat-burning thermogenic supplements, Rebecca was consumed with scheduling her day around her workouts and her sessions at the tanning bed. Rebecca worked out twice a day, monitored her calorie intake religiously and confided in me for extra counseling in an effort to stay on the cutting edge of fat burn. She was perpetually seeking to lower her body fat percentage and to change her appearance. Rebecca was never satisfied and never learned to look in the mirror and accept the things about herself that she couldn't change.

To the bystander, Rebecca was untouchable and confident, so beautiful that she was almost a work of art. To the few who knew her intimately, behind her Gucci clothes and high-end hair extensions, she was a scared little girl. Rebecca had no confidence, no peace and no real joy. The more she perfected her look, the more she spiraled downward internally. I hoped it was a phase of low self-esteem she would outgrow.

One wintry morning, I received a phone call that shook me to the core: Rebecca committed suicide.

She left no explanation other than a short note. The note said that she could continue no longer. In losing Rebecca, the world lost a beautiful mother, a loving wife, and a giving friend. Rebecca was the woman every mother wanted to look like and every man wanted to date. Her physical beauty inspired and captivated all those who surrounded her, and her inner beauty made the people around her feel loved. Tragically, she never saw herself for who she was, and her beauty and life passed her by.

Rebecca's influences on women made me take a new look at the power and role of beauty. Beauty makes people obsess. It is essential to understand that fundamentally, everyone is susceptible to body bumming. It does not discriminate, and allowed to go untreated, can bring devastation upon the least likely characters.

Seven months after Rebecca's unfortunate death, I learned news that another Rebecca in my life attempted suicide. We will call this friend of mine Sandy.

Sandy looked like Barbie, but not in the plastic, over-done way; the money put into Sandy's California look made her look naturally crafted. A warm 30-something party girl, Sandy's beauty drew others to her and her charisma charmed all. Sandy had everything every woman wanted; weekend trips to Cabo, a wealthy and doting husband, three beautiful children, and a perfect body.

Sandy lived a secret life. It is not the kind of secret life you would expect. This secondary lifestyle was not visible to the human eye. Sandy's secret life was her thought life. She battled with extreme depression and could not find contentment. Nothing about her body was ever perfect enough, and she struggled to reconcile these feelings of discontentment.

Sandy had reached a point in her personal journey that life did not have enough beauty, reason or purpose. She concluded that, for her, there was no purpose in continuing. Thankfully though, Sandy is alive. Her attempted suicide failed and she underwent intensive therapy and recovery. Hopefully, in her recovery, she will discover the power of her inner beauty and the freedom that it will provide her.

Like many conventionally stunning people, Sandy had no grasp of her inner or outer beauty. Sandy was confused by her inner identity and the identity assigned to her by the world. She was labeled as someone she didn't see and she felt lost. Life for Sandy became overwhelming when she reached the point that she no longer had the strength to hold onto the waning identity that she was losing on the inside.

Both Sandy and Rebecca gave up on life because their purpose and *joie* in life was too externally focused. These beautiful ladies lived under the microscopic judgment of society; they thrived in the spotlight and were respected based upon their appearance and wealth. While beauty inspires the soul and brings joy to the heart, it must be a combination of the trinity of beauty to truly satisfy the soul. Beauty can be like money in many ways; the more beautiful you are, the more beautiful you feel like you need to be. The more money you have, the more money you need. Be it money or beauty, it can be called greed. Greed can never be satisfied. Moreover, the more dissatisfied you become, the more your insecurities are privy to attack you. Eventually, the onslaught of mental anguish becomes overwhelming and you lose sight of your purpose of existence. It is in this way that Sandy and Rebecca both found themselves considering death.

Don't allow greed to take over the focus of your life, either physically speaking or financially. You will find freedom to live in true happiness. You will find *joie* and the ability to live life at your own rhythm if you just learn to accept who and how you are.

It is important to fully understand the implications and effects of "body depression," as well as our responsibility to ourselves to proactively choose to break free from it. In order to understand our inclinations towards body depression, we must first outline the development of body image in a woman's life:

Women were born into a life of hormonal wonder. This internal roller coaster can influence just about everything in the way we see the world and see ourselves. Some of the hardest challenges women face with body image are oftentimes hormonally magnified. Yes, you will feel more bloated some days more than others simply based on your menstrual cycle. Water retention will impact the scale, how tight your pants fit, the puffiness of your face, the state of your skin and how you feel that day. *Water weight retention can account for five to seven pounds of weight fluctuation on any given day.*

Some days, however, you may just feel down. It's not that you are sad or depressed about something specific or something in your life; rather, you are experiencing body bumming. Body bumming is different from sadness in that you simply feel off for some reason, like a funk. It is like a distant numbing; you struggle to identify it and feel especially uncomfortable in your skin that day.

Body bumming is a transcendent experience of feeling uncomfortably and abnormally out of your skin. It is a level of discomfort that exceeds awkwardness and lends to loathing your physical attributes.

Every woman will inevitably experience the funk of feeling out of place in your own body. How long you wallow in the despair is determined by your own self-will and self-awareness. Some women spend days, months, even years in such a state. Others spend only hours.

Breaking free of body bumming is entirely a mental decision, a choice. Every person will have a different intersection of choices to make. Oftentimes, my crossway is three-fold. When I feel myself getting down, or feeling out of sorts in my own skin, I can choose to exercise the anxiety away, be kind to myself and find my Zen or stay distracted and depressed. Paths one and two, via many tributaries, lead ultimately to self-acceptance. Path three is a treacherous road of disablement.

I have wasted years of my life to distraction. Path three was the most natural pathway for me to wander down, given my type-A personality. The path I and many choose is a battleground of neurosis and freedom. Unfortunately, too many of us take this road, thinking that if we are harsh enough upon ourselves, perhaps, just perhaps, our willpower will triumph and we will finally be content with our bodies. *You cannot force confidence and self-acceptance. You have to choose it.*

The trouble with body dysmorphia is that it is practically impossible for anyone else to understand the depth of pain and mental self-loathing that it causes. Typically, those with distorted body image are their own worst enemy. A mirror can make or break their mood and their entire day. An insecure pear shaped woman might only see the "cottage cheese" on her thighs, she is so caught up in her own mental abuse and self-criticism. She tends to compare herself to everyone she sees and fails to see how others covet her tiny waist and thin upper body. We always want what we don't have.

When your physical body is unhealthily central to your identity, you find yourself living in a field of buried, invisible mines. Every day you fight an uphill battle of loving yourself. If you wake up bloated, your worth is crushed. If your favorite shirt shrunk in the dryer, you convince yourself that you gained weight and that everyone is talking about it behind your back. If you walk by a distorted, unflattering mirror, you are sure that it must be representative of how disgusting others really perceive you to be. And, clearly, if you disgust yourself, how much more worthless must others think you are. Your entire worth as a human being lingers on a string; it hinges on luck in the minefield. The unpredictability of it all strikes so much anxiety into your heart that you lose sight of any other part of your identity.

Since your focus is so intensely fixated on the raw hope that others perceive you as beautiful, you lose yourself entirely. Defining your body image as your identity is like suicide to the soul. By living in fear daily, your perspective on life warps to the point that basic contentment and true joy becomes foreign.

The fitness industry that I work in can be a dangerous zone for those with a sensitive body image. I make my livelihood critiquing other people's physiques, analyzing muscular imbalances, measuring body fat percentage and evaluating peoples' flaws in helping them set their own personal fitness goals. Obviously, there is a positive and a negative approach to my role in the fitness industry, and my decision has the potential to make a very big impact on my own self-image. Once the floodgates of judgment and criticism of any type are opened, I put myself in the line of fire as well. It is like self-flagellation. However, I can choose to approach people with loving eyes, eyes that behold great beauty in each individual. A positive attitude not only affects those around you, but yourself also. I make it my daily purpose to find, appreciate and savor the intricate, unique beauty in everyone I encounter. Doing so frees me into the world of *joie de vivre*.

How, then, do we step away from the self-imposed neurosis to which we are so prone? The only way is by decidedly embarking upon a mental journey of willpower. You must decide to be kind with the words you use to describe yourself, you must think beautiful thoughts about yourself, and you must feign confidence. The body believes what the mind thinks. Thinking confident, beautiful thoughts will transform your true self and free you from your neurotic tendencies.

Think for a moment about how many self-loathing thoughts you allow yourself to think every day. Go ahead, stop and think for five minutes to make an estimate.

Your mind controls your view of life. It is up to you to allow negative thoughts or positive thoughts about yourself dominate your thought pattern and subsequently your life. The direction of your journey is solely in your power.

We attack our own bodies sometimes in the smallest scenarios, so small that we sometimes don't even realize how this act is destroying our esteem from the inside out. Even today, neurotic tendencies and perfectionism still stick to me as thorns in my side. The difference is that I now have the tools to choose a healthier thought pattern. Allow me to share a recent experience that thrust me into this warfare I describe:

A televised appearance as a personal trainer is a coveted opportunity. In fact, when personal trainers start up in the fitness industry, they inevitably have the dream to live, breathe and inspire with such impact that they are classified as "elite trainers" like the ones you see on TV.

A few years ago, my club was highlighted on a CBS morning newscast and two trainers were selected for the spotlight. Like in any profession, there is a hierarchy of personal trainers that, while obviously being based on skills and knowledge to an extent, is mostly based on luck of the draw. A trainer is selected based on location, personality and the idea that they are the all-around trainer and best representative of the gym or company.

To my delighted surprise, I was among the two chosen to appear on live TV at the prime time Monday morning news slot. I was excited, but incredibly anxious the morning of the taping. Even though I had no experience with cameras, acting, or entertaining, I was confident about the actual taping segment and about my ability to wow the crowd. I knew that I could count on personality and charisma to appeal to the audience and I was confident in the workout routine I was going to demonstrate. Here I was, at a huge milestone in my career, and with the opportunity to reach so many more people who needed help, and I was paralyzed by an old enemy. The fear that weighed heavy on my confidence that morning was whether or not I would look fat on TV.

The ten-minute segment was a success. I looked professional, beautiful, and very fit. Confident and pleased, I felt like I had rediscovered myself. It was as if I had pushed the limits of self-discovery to uncover just how extroverted I really am. The news anchor actually applauded me and pulled me aside post-taping to request a second appearance.

I was on cloud nine and was feeling great. I felt especially accomplished in that I was considered to look appropriately fit and toned enough to qualify as a "TV trainer." I was desperate for approval from others to tell me that I was fit enough and beautiful enough to be a top trainer.

When I finally saw the recap internet broadcast of my segment, a self-esteem tragedy ensued. It was only to be expected, since I had cared more about others perception of me, than actually sharing my knowledge and enthusiasm about fitness with the viewers. I hadn't cared what they learned from the segment, only if they thought I was beautiful. Remember, it is as I have said before, the moment you allow others to have more value than yourself as the beholder of your beauty, then that is the moment that you give your self-confidence away. I had set myself up for heartache and panicked body bumming.

My neurosis and self-abusive criticism overwhelmed me like a category five hurricane coming ashore when I watched the internet version of the segment. From the moment the introductory commercial played, I could feel my nerves bubbling up in my stomach, and vulnerability about to be exposed.

Since I had put so much value in what viewers would think of my body, I watched with an expectation to dislike what I saw. When I finally saw myself, I felt like I had been filmed naked. I had subconsciously convinced myself that whatever angles the TV camera caught me at were definitive of my entire existence as a human being.

The moment I saw myself, my heart dropped. No, that wasn't me. That Trish Blackwell looked too short and squatty – yes, I am short, but I am definitely not squatty. In fact, I am petit and cute. Halfway through the segment my shirt flipped out a little and my stomach didn't look as flat as I thought it should have.

My world and my beauty felt like they were coming to end. I felt like a failure. I was disappointed looking at myself. Those couldn't be my shoulders. I look at my arms and shoulders every day at the gym when I train others and work out; mine are strong, toned, beautiful. The ones on TV simply looked big. Never mind that I had been asked back to the studio and been praised excessively by others on how well the segment had gone, no. To me, all that mattered was if I looked skinny.

How, then, do we as women step away from this self-imposed neurosis when it attacks us expectedly or unexpectedly?

I stepped away from it by turning back towards memories of my experience in France. I had to remind myself of the freedom and unconstrained beauty that my French friends exuded and I imagined them watching the TV segment with me. The visualization of their moral support, their praises and their comfort in their skin enabled me to remember that my beauty resides in the core of my being, not in a mirror reflection or in the eye of a video camera. It's amazing: after this mini-escape, I was able to go back and watch the video and to see myself as a whole instead of as a body of divided parts. I looked beautiful, confident, and fit.

We have to remember that sometimes our first impressions of ourselves are not accurate ones. Do not allow these first glimpses to define you, and use positive visualization to weed the criticism out of your mind. This is a journey of mental will power, of kind words and determined thinking on the beauty that is already in you. The more aware we are of the battlefield of the mind, the more victory we will have in our thought lives. The healthier your thought-life, the more *joie de vivre* you will free yourself to enjoy. The choice is yours.

I know I am not alone in such a neurotic struggle. I know, too, that I am not the only one who can break free. You want your misery to go away and to advance in your life, but you constrain yourself out of fear of self-acceptance. You are the only one that holds the keys to your own shackles.

When you are struggling with disordered eating of any type, the fear of regaining weight can be a heavy burden that causes overwhelming anxiety. A recent study published in the International Journal of Eating Disorders (2008; 41, 728-33) found that progressive muscle relaxation, guided imagery and self-directed relaxation were significant contributors to helping disordered eaters achieve a healthy weight. Relaxation techniques, demonstrated by the French lifestyle, show how important rest, balance, and taking time to smell the roses (or whatever your particular Zen is to arrive at your own *joie de vivre*) can be in helping you master loving your skin from the inside out.

Biblical philosophers call the soul the wellspring of living. Artists believe all creative powers are direct reflections of the soul. We admire athletes who put their heart and soul into everything they do. How it is, then, that we squash and snuff out our very own souls?

THE JOURNEY OF BEAUTY AND BODY SHAPE
Skinny, Sexy *à la carte*
L'argent ne fait pas le bonheur.
[Money – or a "perfect" body – doesn't buy happiness.]

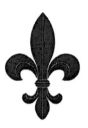

i. Skinny, Sexy SUMMARY:

Living life, like many others things, is a choice. Living is an action, a verb, and therefore, an active choice that we make daily. Beauty is not necessarily something you can capture in a still photograph; rather, it is something in motion, in movement and fully alive.

ii. Skinny, Sexy REFLECTION:

How many days of your life have you been on autopilot rather than actually living according to your heart of hearts? In any given week, how many days do you *live* and how many days do you autopilot yourself? *What do you need to do to "own" and release your beauty?*

iii. Skinny, Sexy PERSONAL APPLICATION:

Learning to be your own beholder begins with looking in the mirror and accepting who you are and the things you cannot change. In accepting the things about yourself that you cannot change, you will discover a newfound peace. With peace comes freedom, and with freedom comes our ability to choose. The power of choice gives you the strength and ability to choose *life* every day.

Fill out the "Twenty Things I love About My Body" section in this chapter. Take your time making the list. Read the list out loud to yourself. Read the list to someone who loves you and refer to the list every time you start feeling down.

iv. Skinny, Sexy EATING:

Resist the temptation to eat when you are feeling bad about your body, for eating in this state of mind will only compound the internal stress you are feeling about yourself already. When you are struggling with body image, distract yourself with something active and physical instead of with food.

v. Skinny, Sexy YOU:

Make a list of all the people in your life that are infused with all three types of beauty. Ask yourself what it is that makes them so attractively different and see if you can emulate their living examples.

Remember, you will find *joie* and the ability to love your body and to live life at your own rhythm if you just learn to accept who and how you are.

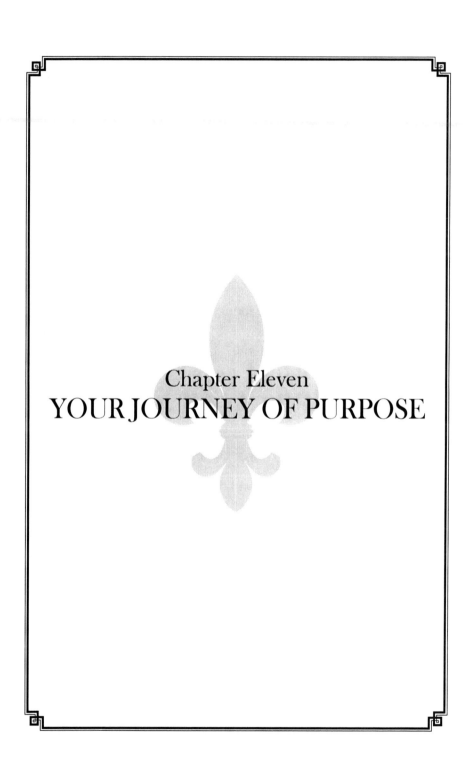

Chapter Eleven
YOUR JOURNEY OF PURPOSE

Chapter Eleven
YOUR JOURNEY OF PURPOSE

In our modern lives of commuting and over-committing, many people feel lost in the day-to-day grind of their lives. They feel this way either because they don't fit the homogenous mold around them or because they are afraid of not being fully accepted by others. Ultimately, our greatest, most paralyzing fear is rejection. Furthermore, we tragically spend much of our lives in self-rejection, which is the ultimate betrayal.

Feeling out of place, awkward, or at risk of being rejected socially can turn into a slippery slope of self-berating. The rejection felt when you don't get the second interview for your dream job, the foolishness you felt when the boy you liked didn't reciprocate your feelings, or the social inadequacy you felt the first time others did not appreciate your efforts at humor, all scar us profoundly.

So we learn from our experiences in which we have suffered pain from making ourselves vulnerable and sharing our most intimate identity. We cower from allowing it to happen again. However, it is in our power to see beauty in these battle wounds of our lives.

The ultimate rejection, though, is when we reject our true selves. I am confident that people feel lost because they are lost in purpose.

If you don't know who you are and what makes you tick, then, yes, you seem to be floating around in stagnancy. You then become no different or more unique than the billions of other humans inhabiting this planet. Nothing is more tragic than this type of self-betrayal; that is, when you reject yourself because you don't yet know yourself. It is no wonder that we have learned to turn to food as a drug or we compensate in the opposite direction and use the control of food to give us a false sense of control over our lives.

I am someone who lived that self-betrayal for the majority of my adolescence; it makes for a lonely life and misunderstood acceptance. Not feeling comfortable in your own skin is the ultimate betrayal of self-rejection. More tragic, however, is the way in which doing so stunts your ability to live the life you were meant to life. We are all here to impact the world and those around us in a very special, very unique way – if you retard and prevent your own self-growth, then you take away what you are truly meant to contribute in this life.

How, then, are we suppose to transition from self-rejection to self-acceptance? It is actually much simpler than we think, and it all starts with the following truth that I learned from my co-worker Alex Kelly-Maartens:

Your body feeds on the thoughts you feed it.

If you hold onto this axiom, you will see that a simple phrase can change everything about your life. AAs Alex Kelly-Maartens, founder of PITAIYO – an exercise discipline that combines Pilates, Tai Chi and Yoga – taught me that for an idea to really impact you, you must own it. You must make it infiltrate every aspect of what you do, make it what you eat, what you breathe, and what you think. Kelly-Maartens' class is based on the concept for which the PITAIYO acronym represents: "Put it together all in your orbit." She coaches her students on what, in my opinion, every American should learn and own: that you have control of what you put into your orbit. You can create your own positive orbit or negative orbit, and the influence of that orbit will affect every aspect of your life if you allow it to.

In following the example of PITAIYO, you can make a simple phrase and change your entire existence. In being aware of what is in your orbit, you will not only change the way you live, but you will change the lives of others around you.

Think about Kelly-Maartens' philosophy again: *"your body feeds on the thoughts you feed it."* The statement highlights the fact that we are, by nature, hungry creatures. Our stomachs provide the most carnal, superficial hunger we experience. We have a deeper hunger in our souls, though, one that many of us try to ignore. Our minds and our entire being are starving for something purposefully substantial and filling. It is an innate desire that is part of our construction as human beings. We hunger for the truth of our identity, for a firm understanding as acting affirmation on our purpose of existing and our beauty as individuals.

Unbeknownst to even our closest friends, many of us are hopelessly insecure. When the dominating factor of your thought life is focused on your physical appearance or on others' perception of you, then your body will feast on the same. Even some of the most successful people in the world are hopelessly insecure. The wealthy are paranoid that they are only liked for their money, the famous fear that they are being used for publicity, and the beautiful are frightened that when their looks fade they will be a disappointment. We are afraid of not measuring up and of not fitting in. We are no more mature than when we first experienced social interaction and favoritism between friends on our first day at school as kindergarteners.

I confess that I, too, have fed my body mean, self-abusive criticism. I have spoon fed my mind thoughts of needing to be thinner, needing to be taller, and needing to be more voluptuously proportioned. I convinced myself that those were "needs" to complete my beauty, and the moment that my mind chose that instrumental word of "need," the focus of my life shifted. What my mind defined as a "need" became my purpose for living.

Subsequently, the thoughts I thought about myself were cruelly judgmental, blatantly harsh, and at the center of my thought-life.

How could they not be, when I mentally classified the achievement of physical perfection as a "need" for my personal happiness? It is no surprise that my body fed upon the lies I lived in my mind.

It cannot be exaggerated: your mind lies. If you lie to yourself, your mind will lie to you. To break free of body-rejection, you must first recognize that the thoughts you have trained your mind to think are not true. Until you can commit to having the discipline of mind to weed out years of negative, self-abusive thoughts and to qualify them as lies, then you will remain a prisoner in a state of numb existence.

It is no surprise that I struggled for years with a distorted body image; I spent most of my life being my own worst enemy. When I look into a mirror, I still have to weed out the first thoughts that come to mind, because, you see, they still attack me.I lied to myself for almost ten years; it will take time for me to fully retrain my instinctive thought patterns, but if I know the truth and hold onto the truth, then the truth will set me free. One day I know that I will be able to look in the mirror and see only beauty. It's just like the French say; we do age fine in beauty, like a fine wine.

It is here that I have a choice. I can choose to continue to subscribe to the years of lies and disappointment towards my body, or I can choose freedom. It is a harder decision than one would think, because change is scary. Oftentimes we concede to thought patterns because, well, we've always thought like that, and we just resign to thinking that it's simply the way we are programmed. I implore you to consider your mind as wine – it is always aging and getting better.

Remember this: your body will morph into what you allow it to be in your mind. If you think you look bloated or frumpy in a mirror one day, then you have opened the floodgates to a day of bloated frustration. Negative thoughts will reign in your mind all day. You will actually begin to feel however you told yourself you look. It's true; think about a time in your past that you felt fat in the mirror – did you not feel a bit more self-conscious or as if clothes fit tighter for the rest of the day? Or another time when your face was broken out – did you feel like an awkward adolescent and it seemed like no one looked you in the eyes but stared at your unsightly skin instead?

The moment you judge yourself is the moment you give permission for others to do the same. In the moment that your mind chooses a reactive thought to an image you see, that instantaneous microsecond of a moment is your opportunity to control your destiny. This is the moment we must all train to be aware of and to be disciplined to control.

Body hang-ups also ensue as a cop-out and distraction for anxiety-producing circumstances in life. For example, my best friend in Chicago admitted to me recently that she has been besieged by the stress that her battle with body image has upon her life. This is a struggle that she shares with no one; not even her family is aware of her perverted relationship with food or of the impact is has on her life. It is worth being said here that she is an unexpected candidate for disordered eating and poor body image. She is a tall blonde, gregarious with confidence and humor that attracts people to her with a magnetic effect. Her slender build, chic understanding of fashion, and success in the corporate hustle of Chicago make her the "it" girl of her elite social circle. She is one of the most talented, sincere, and loyal people I have ever met. However, she is not able to see the joy that she brings to so many. She cannot see it because she does not know herself well enough yet.

Recently, her darkest moments of body-bumming have been coinciding with the ups and downs of her current relationship; the moment she opens herself emotionally to be fully vulnerable with her lover, she panics and reverts back to either binging or purging, both of which leave her feeling lousy, unworthy, and unlovable. Subconsciously, she has fed her mind thoughts of disgrace and shame, and the focus on her existence is directed solely to finding perfection in her physical appearance. If he rejects her or ever betrays her, she will blame it on imperfections of her body, or on her paralyzing distraction and selfishness of her bulimia. Otherwise, any rejection is fundamentally a rejection of the most intimate part of her, her true self. Such fear of rejection is almost too confusing and too scary to consider, so we create our own obstacles and fortresses of protection. It is literally a fight for survival, a fight to love your body or to love yourself.

My dear friend has not be yet able to convince herself that she can love both her body and herself or that she can be loved for both. She believes that to be true, but she hasn't mastered living it to be true.

So then, how do people master living a truth that they believe in their heart but haven't yet convinced their mind to follow in such faith? It starts with training the subconscious with positive thoughts and allowing the mind and body to pursue the innate *joie* they already possess. This can distinguish the difference between living half heartedly and whole-heartedly. If we can live with our whole hearts, then we will be able to fully pursue our life's purpose.

Love your body *and* love yourself. This seems simple enough, but is a great challenge.

Think about the people in your life. Of those that you can confidently say love their body, would you say that they are also confident in themselves? Do they rely on their looks as their identity? Where do they find their self-worth? Can you actually list and name these individuals? If so, write their names in the table provided. Next to their names, try to find three qualities about that person that makes him or her stand out so in your mind. Take the qualities you admire in them as lesson for your heart. Remember, we are drawn to the people in our lives that we are meant to learn and grow from. Nothing is an accident.

CONFIDENT PEOPLE IN MY LIFE:

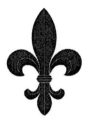

1. _____

2. _____

3. _____

4. _____

5. _____

I know an overwhelming number of "confident" people that cling to the superficiality of their appearance because that is what is praised by society. They are confident in the English sense of the word, but definitely not by French definition. They are praised and accepted for what they look like and are afraid of the emptiness of soul that such praise makes them feel on the inside. I once dated a runway and magazine model who turned out to be more internally insecure than he was externally beautiful. It all goes back to the old saying that one shouldn't judge a book by its cover. We cannot allow ourselves to believe that external beauty always means internal beauty, nor is it at all related to true happiness.

Please don't mistake my words: these people are not in the least empty on the inside, but they have never had to search out their identity since society has handed it to them based upon their looks. Those who love their bodies in this fashion are desperately insecure and sometimes afraid to dig deep in order to discover their heart of hearts, all out of fear that they might be disappointed in what they find.

THE CHOICE OF GARDENINING YOUR MIND AND BODY

Unfortunately, the vast majority of Americans neither love their bodies nor themselves. We all want to make a difference in this world, but we sometimes just don't know how. We are blind to seeing that if we are just true to the deepest desires of our true being, then we will make a tremendous impact by just being vibrantly alive and vibrantly ourselves. It is a natural desire to want to make a difference, because it has been programmed into the makeup of our being. We are so afraid that we will fail to make the impact that weighs heavily on the destiny of our hearts that many of us just stop bothering to connect with both ourselves and others.

Those of us who have begun a journey of identity discovery and purposeful living have begun to learn to love ourselves. Be wary, however, to not become too distracted to take the time to self-reflect and remember who you really are. Staying true to yourself and your purpose is a continual process, a daily endeavor and one that is guided by *joie.*

Once you learn *who* you are, you have to learn *how* to love yourself. Then, you have to learn how to love your body. Loving your body necessitates cultivating a mantra of self-acceptance and understanding. It is a gardening of the mind that results in a gardening of the body as well.

How many of us neither love our bodies nor love ourselves? It saddens me to say that I think many Americans fall into such classification and don't even know it. Allow me to clarify: I am not saying here that the majority of our nation is walking around with their heads down, in oversized t-shirts and with a do-nothing attitude for themselves. I am asserting that most of our nation is numb. We are numb to ourselves. Most of us keep ourselves so busy that we don't even know what emotions we feel, let alone *who* we are as people. To genuinely love yourself, you must know yourself. To make an impact on the world, you must know yourself.

If you don't know yourself, you cannot share yourself. Not sharing yourself with the world is selfish. Many of us live selfish lives not because we are selfish at heart, but because we are foolishly fearful. It is a fear of betrayal, of rejection, and of not having any real potential to make an impact on others.

We choose instead to numb ourselves and live in lonely cocoons of insecurity. Living in insecurity is like trying to run with a ball and chain around your ankle. We are either selfishly obsessed with our appearances, or are selfishly guarded with our true selves. Neither of these approaches are constructive ways for an individual to fulfill his or her purpose for existing.

If you want to get out of the rut of thinking only about yourself, in whatever capacity controls you, then it is time for you to discover your purpose for existing.

What is your life calling? What are the quirks, the interests, the gifts you were given that combine to create a unique contribution to the world? What is it that makes you tick, and how can you share that with others? When you think about these things, think about everything that you enjoy, from small things to bigger things. Think about hobbies, think about dreams, think about careers, think about every element of your life and being.

I decided that my purpose on Earth is to make others around me feel valued. I want to inspire others to love more: to love themselves, to love their bodies, to love others, and to love life more. In what I do and how I live, I want to be a motivator and encourager. I want to be unapologetically myself and authentically sincere with everyone whom I encounter. I love roller coasters, I love running, I love writing, I love learning new languages, I love everything French, and I especially love laughing.

What mark do you want to leave on others? What words do you want others to use to describe you? What legacies are you are going to leave behind you?

The legacies you choose to develop are either going to leave a positive or negative impact on those you whom you love. Obviously, we all want to leave a positive legacy, but how many of us really do? Positivity must seep through everything you do. Live, breathe, and think positivity and you will find that the world around you will change and your purpose will expand.

Some say that choosing to be positive is a daily choice. I disagree. It is a moment to moment choice. Some days, you may have to re-center your mind hourly. Other days, you may fight minute by minute. Ultimately, the most important thing to remember is that you do have control; you have the final say, and you – only you – have the ability to feed your mind healthy thoughts.

Healthy thoughts produce a healthy body. Your mind must be cultivated like a garden. Create a garden of healthy thoughts in your mind and learn to nurture and tend them through to full maturity and fruition. As in a garden, you never just grow one thing, and you never have a garden for just one season. Gardening of the mind is a perpetual act, with different types of care demanded with each changing season. A garden is sown, watered, weeded, nourished, protected, and pruned. It is watched with patience and with a discerning eye for intruders. It is protected and tended to with the care that a mother lends to her child. Patience in gardening is essential, but so is a vision of hope in what is to come.

Gardening is about making something come out of nothing into full life and vibrancy. Maybe that is why I was so moved by urban gardens. Our minds are like cities in that they need to be sprinkled with gardens to enable life to truly thrive. We need the gardens as escapes from the city life we are confined to in our minds. Bursting with life and greens, they are places where our hearts and souls find revival. They are places where nature can speak to us and give us life.

Planting a garden is only half the battle. Successful gardening requires meticulous maintenance. So too, in gardening the mind, planting positive thoughts is only half the battle – positivity must be maintained and cultivated on a daily basis. When the buds of the flowers start to peep through, all the attention you have mindfully paid your garden will be worth double its time. You will have ownership of your garden and pride for how you controlled its development. You will be able to share your harvest to empower them.

I never liked gardens before I went to France. After my first stroll through the Parisian *Jardins de Luxembourg* I knew that what I was experiencing in that moment was unlocking my soul in a way I never knew possible. I can still recall entering the garden gates unknowingly on my second day in Paris, giggling with my best friend Melissa who was exploring with me, and suddenly becoming speechless as we walked. Luxembourg was like a hidden oasis brimming with green life inside the grey stone city walls of the narrow Parisian streets. The August breeze kept us cool in the heat of the sun as we walked through a world unbeknownst to us. Watercolor artists painted in the shade of the lily-covered ponds, young children pushed wooden sailboats around the central fountains and joggers trotted aimlessly along the dirt pathway that intersected throughout the entirety of the garden. I felt peace and I felt alive. It was that day, while sitting in the grass surrounded by lovers and picnickers, that – as film director Alexander Payne said in the short the *14ème Arrondissemont* in the film *Paris, Je t'Aime* – "I fell in love with Paris and Paris fell in love with me."

During my time in Paris, and every time I have gone back since, the *Jardins de Luxembourg* are the soul of my stay. Even if I am only able to spend five minutes there, it is all I need to remind my soul of how it feels to come alive. *Les Jardins de Luxembourg, les Touleries, Vaux-le-Vicompte*, and of course, *Versailles* enabled me to experience indescribable transcendence through manicured nature. These French gardens speak like art to my being and soul, and like art, they are fragile and demand maintenance.

Gardening creates a unique sense of accomplishment for its creator; it is a sense that encompasses both immediacy and patience. It brings life. Interestingly enough, gardening is a constant. It is never finished; every season brings new growth and new weeds.

The mind is no different; we must be in a continual state of self-awareness and self-evaluation to properly cultivate the full potential of the gardens of our mind and soul. For those of us who have made getting "skinny" or achieving our "perfect weight" the focus of our minds, there is a seed you must plant in your garden to find your way to freedom.

The skinny, sexy mind seed: the only way to getting skinny and sexy is to find another purpose for living.

You have to arrive at a point in your gardening that you believe that the extra plump squash you grow is no less beautiful or worthy than the narrow, skinny squash you harvest. Too many of us who struggle with body identity arrive at a crossroads where we tend to get stuck: we try to make our garden look exactly like the garden of our neighbor. We forget too easily that every garden is a work of art and beautifully unique in its own way. Our bodies are the same. We wallow in the pit of body rejection because we are so obsessed and distracted with achieving our idea of the perfect body that we have no other purpose for living. I am ashamed and relieved to admit that I too have been guilty of this.

My purpose for living for almost ten years had been to find conventional beauty in myself according to media standards and expectations. In total, I have wasted countless months of my life obsessing over approximately three pounds. I obsessed and allowed myself to get depressed over an extra centimeter of skin on my stomach, a half-inch of skin on my inner thighs, and a broad bone structure that blessed (or I thought had cursed) me with an athletic build. My battle with disordered eating and self-hatred was fundamentally a battle over a few extra centimeters of skin and a few pounds. Essentially, I allowed less than five pounds to steal my *joie de vivre* for ten years.

That is no exaggeration; it is a life-altering realization. Usually it is something minutely small and seemingly innocent that steals life from us without notice. We don't even realize it is happening before it is too late. With that in mind, what is it in your life that is stealing your ability to live with *joie?*

I had been so distracted with my imperfections that I questioned men's attraction to me. I feared that I was good looking enough or good enough of an example of physical health to go into personal training, and I turned down hundreds of social invitations out of fear of how I would look in clothes that night. I chose to be alone and I distrusted anyone close to me. When I looked at myself in the mirror, all I could see were my flaws, and I assumed that that was all anyone else saw as well. When you look in the mirror, what do you see first? Whatever it is that you see, you must take time to reflect upon what that actually means to your body image and confidence.

How many days, months, or years of your life have you selfishly and so foolishly wasted like I did? Be honest with yourself. How many?

Permit me to be the one to tell you that life is better than that. I have lived it on both sides. The days I describe above were days of misery and loneliness. The ones I am living now are days of freedom, awareness, *joie* and true living. I am now living with a *skinny, sexy* mind, and living in this way is *good.*

It is time to embark upon the journey of re-training your mind. Do you believe that you are just as beautiful twenty pounds heavier than you are now? You must believe that you are beautiful no matter the size or shape you may be. Stop allowing the physical circumstances of your body to steal away the rest of your life. Stop allowing it to steal the joy you have to share with the world. Stop being self-centered and commit yourself to disciplining your mind.

Put positive, loving thoughts into your orbit and see what happens. You will be surprised how easy it will be to overcome the years of lies your mind has fed you. Feed your body good thoughts, keep your blinders on as to what others are doing around you and simply control your orbit and your orbit alone. Garden your mind with positivity and live life to the beat of your own rhythm. The rest will take care of itself.

THE JOURNEY OF PURPOSE
Skinny, Sexy *à la carte*
Qui cherche, trouve.
[Seek and ye shall find.]

i. Skinny, Sexy SUMMARY:

The ultimate rejection in the journey of purpose is when we reject our true selves. If you don't know who you are and what makes you tick, then, yes, you seem to be floating around in stagnancy. Nothing is more tragic than this type of self-betrayal; that is, when you reject yourself because you don't yet know yourself.

We are all here to impact the world and those around us in a very special, very unique way – if you retard and prevent your own self-growth, then you take away what you are truly meant to contribute in this life.

ii. Skinny, Sexy REFLECTION:

Your body feeds on the thoughts you feed it. *What thoughts do you feed your body?* How many days, months, or years of your life have you selfishly and foolishly wasted on hating your imperfections?

iii. Skinny, Sexy PERSONAL APPLICATION:

If you want to accept your body with confidence and love, you must first recognize that the thoughts you have trained your mind to think are not true. Make a list of the negative things you have told yourself about your body, about your personality and about what you can and cannot do. Complete the list, and then rip it up. Rip it into as many pieces as you can and throw them all away. You are no longer that person or those negative thoughts. You are perfect just the way you are.

iv. Skinny, Sexy EATING:

Allow yourself some grace in your eating habits. Refuse to allow guilt to partake in your meals with you and start making conscientious choices for petit splurges to complement your new healthy, natural, balanced eating.

v. Skinny, Sexy YOU:

The skinny, sexy mind seed of success is that the only way to getting skinny and sexy is to find another purpose for living. Put positive, loving thoughts into your orbit and see what happens. Make a list of your new skinny, sexy, positive, and purposeful thoughts and keep it in your wallet so that you can frequently remind yourself of your great worth.

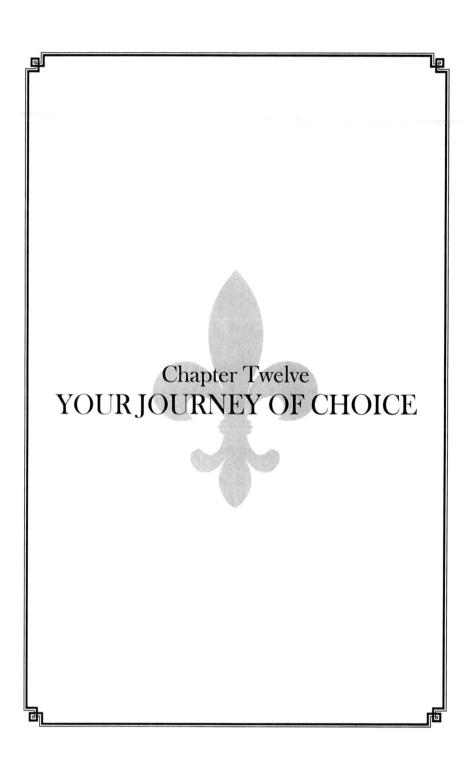

Chapter Twelve
YOUR JOURNEY OF CHOICE

Chapter Twelve
YOUR JOURNEY OF CHOICE

There is a metaphorical bridge in our lives that can be one of the most important bridges we cross in our entire existence. We choose to cross the bridge or we choose not to. It is a treacherous drawbridge that is both inviting and threatening. We yearn to cross it though we subconsciously live in fear of falling off and regretting the effort. This bridge is the bridge of self-discovery; it is the bridging of our self-acceptance between the formative experiences of our childhood and our true adult identity. It is the moment in which we decide to identify and accept our true selves or to condemn ourselves to the stains of our past.

The glaring stain of my personal past and journey of self-discovery is an eating disorder. What is yours?

The waters underneath this crossway can be a mix of murky depths and turbulent bellows. All who attempt the path of self-discovery fear that ultimately they will fall back into old habits and old identities, and find themselves trapped again in the waves of depression and stagnancy. Or, perhaps, even worse, the ultimate disappointment: discovery that we have nothing truly special about us at the core of our nature.

Crossing the bridge of self-awareness is scary. There are many reasons why people subconsciously choose not to cross the bridge. Some fear never being understood by others, while some fear not making a difference with their lives. Most of us are simply afraid of discovering that we are just *average.* We live in a lonely cynicism cushioned by faded memories of worn off childhood fairytales. As a whole, we feel lost in life. The adult reality of living is lonely and confusing and as a result, many of us tend to stick to the easiest, most direct life path we can find. Long gone is the innocent belief we were taught as children that we can do *anything* we want. Much forgotten is how easily we believed in ourselves and in bedtime stories that made us believe we were modern day versions of beautiful princesses or world heroes. We knew we were special as children but we have allowed the cynicism of the world to taint us. We find it easier to wallow in the comfort of the negative known, than dare re-explore the joyful, (some may say naïve) thinking of our youth. We settle, and then years go by and we wonder why we feel like we're missing out on the good life of truly living. Many people experience a glimpse back into the good life through travel, though they struggle to incorporate the freedom and *joie* they experience while vacationing into their everyday lives.

The good life is in our own hands. Allow yourself to travel back to the innocence of your youth: you can do *anything* you set your mind to. At what point in your maturity did you lose grasp on that fundamental life truth? Who was it in your life that made you feel silly and immature for daring to hold on to a personal dream of yours or to the belief that you are unstoppable in your determination?

It is time to go back to the basics. True discovery of self lies in the simplest of questions: what is the one thing in the world that you most want to do or achieve?

Your answer to that question will guide you to a domino-like discovery of what you most deeply yearn for and desire in your heart of hearts. You are uniquely crafted and gifted to fulfill your dreams; you must believe fundamentally that there is a reason that you possess certain desires, interests, and passions. Identifying the things in your life that make your heart come alive is the first step to truly coming alive.

Secondly, you must acknowledge that we are creatures in continual change and we have the amazing ability to control how we change and develop. We are not a product of our circumstances; we are a product of our choices.

The power of development lies entirely in our minds and is dependent on what thoughts we choose to think. Remember, we are what we think. If you think that you are just "average," then you will be just average. If you are confident that you have something great that only you can contribute to the world and to those around you in your way of joyful living, then you will be a magnetic personality whom those around you aspire to mimic. *Nothing draws admiration more than authenticity.* Authenticity of self cannot come without crossing the bridge and identifying your heart of hearts.

Within your heart of hearts, you must hold strong. There is a difference between believing in yourself, and confidently pursuing your passions with the certainty that you will succeed. How, if you are following your heart, could you ever doubt that you will not be successful? Why are we fearful of failure if we are living life whole-heartedly? It is impossible to fail if you live by the interests of your heart.

This, however, is where mental strength is of the utmost importance. The essence of confidently living in joy is grounded in your ability to hold on to the essence of who *you* are individually as a human being. Every thought you think directs you somewhere; it is impossible to coast through your experience of life without being propelled by your thought life. You are either thinking thoughts that point you to fulfilling your purpose on Earth, or you are thinking negatively and are directing yourself towards numbing the vibrancy of your individualism.

Thinking [and repeating it daily] something as simplistic as the phrase *"I am strong"* can have a tremendous impact on your entire life. In such a statement you recognize that you have physical strength, muscle tone, mental and emotional fortitude, and an ability to protect yourself. Ultimately, this physical strength that you feel and recognize in yourself serves as a catalyst in solidifying your emotional and mental strength. Thoughts are like dominos, they become interconnected whether you like it or not and they affect every part of every aspect of you.

In disciplines that focus on training the connection between the mind and the body, the ability of the mind to be refined is of the utmost importance. Kelly-Maartens has an incredible ability to refocus the mind on positive thinking. In class, she instructs participants to visualize and meditate on the phrase *"I am strong"* while holding a yoga pose. You are what you think, Alex proclaims as she urges her class to hold strong to that short mantra for the entire week.

I took on her challenge and committed to repeating the token phrase, *I am strong*, out loud ten times a day for a week to see how my subconscious would react. Sure enough, Monday morning my subconscious recalled it naturally. Monday afternoon during a workout, my mind automatically started repeating it and I felt stronger and more confident in my ability to finish what I was doing. Alex is right: You *are* what you think. It really can't get any simpler than that, and that is why so many French are confident. They are culturally raised to think themselves confident. I know this because I spent over a year with French children and maturing adolescents. They grow to think themselves into what they want to be and they do not fear the judgment of others simply because criticism is not as infiltrated into the culture as it is here in the States.

It is now your time to set the dominos up to fall your way and think yourself into who you are meant to be. Choose to be confidently you. Choose to say, "I *am* sexy." The dominos will begin to tip, and you will like what you see and feel.

I once attended a personal training conference where a speaker taught me one of the most beautifully simplistic truths I could ever speak to myself. As an ice-breaker for his presentation, he had everyone in the room, which was a room of over two hundred very fit personal trainers, stand up, put their arms around one another's shoulders, and proclaim in unison:"I am *sexy*! I am *smart*, and I am *strong*!"

It was amazing how uncomfortable many of the participants were in saying such a statement out loud. I even met trainers that confessed later that they didn't have the courage to mutter the words, that they were too embarrassed, or that they just felt too silly to participate. Need I repeat that this was an audience of intelligent, professional, and chiseled certified personal trainers? How could they, of all populations, be uncomfortable saying such a power phrase?

Like the group of insecure personal trainers, it is as if we all sit around waiting for someone to choose our destiny and identity for us. We want others to tell us that we are successful. We as trainers want to be recognized by others for our extreme physiques and our ability to motivate. We all yearn to be told that we are beautiful. Why, though, do we need others to tell us what we already know?

It is time to step out of your comfort zone. Stop sitting around and waiting for affirmation from others, and give it to yourself. You and only you have the ability to choose who you are and to choose to live fully.

There is a difference between choosing confidence and pretending to be confident. You must be honest with yourself, with the wounds of your past, and with the things that make your heart come alive. Do not pretend to be something that you are not for that will only hinder your quest for living. Do not be something that someone else wants you to be, be who you want to be. Whatever you do, don't lie to yourself about this one thing. I know too many people who pretend that they are happy or confident and who, once you peel away the layers of pain, are actually caught up in a cycle of self-hatred. Some folks cross a road where giving up on themselves is easier than pushing through the pain of self-discovery. I know countless women who have stayed in an unhealthy, loveless relationship because they are afraid that they will find no one else to love them and the few extra pounds of curves they carry with them. Weight can weigh on someone's self-worth and esteem so profoundly that they are unable to identify themselves as anything but sub-par, though, to the world, they profess being happy and comfortable with themselves. They harbor a secret that they feel is safe with no one. Such secret-keepers will never avoid the inevitable. The need for self-awareness is crucial to true understanding of your identity and to true *joie de vivre*.

Janet, like many of us, is afraid of being average. She is a successful personal trainer with a magnetic personality that makes everyone around her feel at home. Just being around Janet and her authenticity makes you feel just a little bit more whole and more confident in just being you. She has a unique gift with people.

Janet was one of the trainers unable to proclaim "I am *sexy*! I am *smart*, and I am *strong*!" because she thinks she is a Plain Jane. Though she is the farthest thing from it, her eyes see what her mind has told her, and for years she has believed that she was just the All-American, average country girl. She describes her stylish blonde bob as flat and frumpy, while I've over-heard people referring to her as "the girl with the perfect hair." People are magnetically drawn to Janet because she is simply unapologetically herself. She accepts where she came from and she incorporates her family into every aspect of her life. Warm and welcoming to others, it is practically impossible to be around Janet without laughing or feeling at home. She is authentically sincere and one of the most trustworthy people I have met in my life. I speak from experience that Janet's receptive smile and warmth can literally be a lifesaver to a person in a period of depression. Like I said, Janet has a gift.

The interesting thing about Janet is that she doesn't know she has that gift. The disconnect that can occur in the psyche between reality and between your own self-perception is amazing. Janet lets her past wear her down. It didn't happen all at once, but slowly, over time, subconsciously. Years of random family members not believing in her, arbitrary comments on her choice to pursue her education, and a buildup of painful memories of not being properly recognized for effort and achievement in the past have become her burden. It is a burden that she is fighting desperately to lift off her shoulders. It is a burden that she must free herself from before fully making it across the bridge.

Like Janet, many of us tend to undermine our best qualities and personality traits. We assume that everyone has the same strengths we do (making us technically "average") and that, at the end of the day, we are therefore no better than average people. We yearn to be someone special, but fundamentally we feel ridiculous thinking such a thought, so we protect ourselves behind a self-belittling nature.

We tend to allow the people and experiences of our lives to shackle us to the past. Unfortunately, all too often, the people that shape our life vision are the ones involved in our most tragic moments of development. It is up to you to make sure these people help you shape your vision positively and in the right direction.

I call these people and tragic moments the arrows of the past. The people whose arrows wound you tend to be the people in your life that understand you best. Likewise, such people feel entitled to share their opinion and guidance since they have walked with you along your life-path previously.

I urge you to be careful who you trust with your heart. The heart is the wellspring of living, and you will dry out your own hearts' well if you allow too many other influences to dominate the true desires of your heart. Only you are able to know what deep desires make you uniquely you. Allowing other people to over-influence you is the best way to deny yourself personal growth. I see it repeatedly in both myself and my clients; when you live your life to please others, you will always feel inadequate and disappointed.

Invasion of the heart is most often committed by the negative people in your life. It must never been forgotten that jealousy makes people do awful things. Oftentimes, the negative players in our lives that weigh us down are cynics who are simply just disappointed in the unfolding of their own lives. So focused on the negative and on how terribly difficult life is, these glass-half-empty people are afraid to move past the past, and they subsequently do their best to scare everyone else around them to stay there with them.

No one wants to be alone. It only makes sense that, on a subconscious level, those that live in cynical fear yearn to bring others into misery with them. A negative person never allows themselves to move forward, to cross the bridge, because they are more comfortable in the known than in the unknown and uncontrollable. They are able to control their negativity, but live in fear of being disappointed or hurt. Rather than take the risk, negative people feel safer staying discontent in the past.

It is now your job to recognize the negative players in your life. Filter them out; think about the ways in which they influence and impact your thought-life, and cleanse yourself by noticing how stagnating they are in their own development. It is your choice whether or not you listen to them and whether or not you will continue to allow them to prevent you from crossing the bridge of self discovery. It is up to you to seek out balanced counsel in the wise and compassionate people who you admire in your life.

Do you want to stay in unsettled complacency or do you want to experience the endless joys of the real experience of living and *joie*? In the film *Braveheart,* William Wallace grasped the essence of this vital truth.At the climax of the movie, Wallace inspires courage in his troops by reminding them of the essence of human nature, proclaiming: "Every man dies, but not every man really lives!" Be one of those men, or women, that really live. It is up to you. It all comes back to a choice.

Now that you have recognized the wound-lickers in your life, I want you to think of the five women or men in your life that you admire. Make a list; come up with five. These are people who are beautifully confident, powerful in who they are, and unapologetically themselves. They are the people who inspire you to be a better version of yourself.

MY FIVE POWER PEOPLE:

1. _____

2. _____

3. _____

4. _____

5. _____

Spend five minutes thinking about each one of these role models and identify the traits that stand out and draw you to them. Be specific. The more specific you are, the more you will learn and grow. We admire what we want to be. Use your admiration for positive self-nourishment and development.

TRAITS I ADMIRE & ASPIRE TO HAVE:

1. _____

2. _____

3. _____

4. _____

5. _____

I am convinced that people cross paths for a reason. We are meant to learn from every single person who is placed into the pathways of our lives. However, if we don't take the time to slow down and actually observe what it is about the people in our lives that we admire or love so much, then we miss the reason why they were brought into our lives in the first place. Record the list of traits that you admire and add it to your own personal list of qualities that you would like to have.

There is great value in remembering that by simply meditating on a quality you would like to have, you will start to develop it yourself. I mimicked the French to the best of my ability while I lived in France. I embraced every aspect of French culture seemingly possible, and at the end of the day, I developed French qualities. The same can be said of a pose in a yoga class. As you wobble around, struggling to gain balance during the pose, you may, naturally, get frustrated and begin to huff and puff yourself into giving up. Or, you may repeat softly to yourself: "I am patient," and you will find that your body will respond accordingly. Tense muscles will relax, a racing mind will focus, and time will seem like it is standing still. *You are what you think.* Similarly, you can gather a harvest of virtues simply by desiring to do so. The following virtues are attainable by virtue of the mind and willingness of self: good listening skills, empathy, genuine enthusiasm for others, kindness, patience, love, faith, and sincerity. You can also think your way to better body posture, self-confidence, and self-respect.

The women in my life whom I admire are power-women. They walk around with their shoulders back, chest out and chin up. They look people directly in their eyes and they are comfortable walking into a room of strangers and striking up a conversation. Leaders, they command respect and admiration from all who surround them. Their confidence emanates like sunshine on a summer day, people are attracted to their positive aura and their ability to listen. I find each of the women I look up to so uniquely beautiful that I do not aspire to look like them. Rather, I hope to someday act like them, for I know that it is their full balance of beauty that makes them so outstanding.

I have made a decision to fully know myself and to love what I know. What will it take for you to make that decision for yourself?

Not loving your body, every inch of the skin you are in, prevents you from fully loving and knowing yourself. This internal fight for reconciliation can dominate your thought life. The result is that you become so focused on the physical that you miss out on real living and real growth.

CHOOSING TO LOVE
YOURSELF NAKED

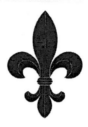

You can control your destiny with simple pleasures and a determined mind. As Kelly-Maartens taught us, put it all together in your orbit. Live what you believe; be positive in word and thought. Create an environment, or orbit, that welcomes all shapes, sizes, colors, and abilities. Allow yourself to be part of that orbit in your own mind. Once you have found the freedom of exhilaration in mind, body and soul this concept can provide, you will be able to savor the *petites plaisirs* in life. The *petites plaisirs* make the world go round and they, if properly embraced, can help you love your body.

Among the lessons France entrusted to me, one of the most poignant in forming my *skinny, sexy mind* was France's openness towards nudity. I am not speaking specifically of nude sunbathing, as that is more generally a European practice, and not specifically French. Rather, it is something naturally and beautifully embedded in the culture.

Any traveler in France will notice the difference in advertisements on TV, on billboards and in magazines. It is normal to see breasts, couples mid-copulation, and naked bodies. However, my freedom in my skin came from some personal instances I experienced while working in Périgueux.

It was required for all teachers to get a yearly physical, so one afternoon I walked to my neighborhood physician's building. After a very confusing amount of paperwork and blood work, I was escorted for my check-up and then for a gynecological exam. Each station where I was led for the check-up was staffed by a different doctor. When I entered the OBGYN section, the male doctor and female nurse closed the door, and asked me to undress and to sit down on the examination table. I was certain I had mistranslated their instructions and asked them to repeat themselves. I looked around for the hospital robe or cover-up I expected them to give me and saw nothing. They both stared at me impatiently, so I undressed to my birthday suit and sat on the cold medal examination table. Without blushing, the doctor pushed my body back on the table, lifted my legs into the examination stirrups and proceeded with his job, a little bothered that I had been so modest and hesitant.

My *Trépied* partner in crime, Angi, had a similar experience, though she was asked to do the entire check-up in the nude. Angi, who is very well-endowed, walked around holding herself and every doctor fussed at her for doing so because it was slowing down their examination time. Angi remembers walking from room to room totally naked and thinking to herself how freeing it was and how such a phenomenon would never happen in America. In France a body is a body and it doesn't always have to be hidden. Also, when the body is exposed, it doesn't always have to be sexual. In our French medical experiences, there was no room for modesty and in fact, body confidence was almost forced on us. The looks we got from the French doctors and nurses when we hesitated to undress was enough to make anyone want to be free in their skin, too. It was as if they were saying, "bof, so what if you have a little bit of tummy" or, "so what if you feel a little bloated today," and it was at that point in my journey that I realized that the body doesn't need to be hidden the way we hide it in America.

Another novel approach to nudity is found in French locker rooms. While in Périgueux, I competed for the local swim team, the A.S.P.T.T Equipe de Natation. We traveled around France competing against other teams in meets. I went to one championship meet in Libourne where instead of medals, we were awarded magnum bottles of regional wine, and I even had the opportunity to compete and place in the French National Championships in Bordeaux.

The experience in the pool was no different from anything a swimmer would experience in America, but everything else surrounding it was totally foreign. In America, swimmers are known to be very open about their bodies since they practically live in their bathing suits and are as close to naked as you can get in public America. In France, it took me a few days to get over the shock of what I experienced with my teammates in the locker rooms. In France, there are no individual changing rooms or shower stalls. My teammates would simply strip off their clothes, be naked and talk in groups while they finally got to putting on their bathing suits. If someone walked into the locker room and needed to greet someone naked, there was no hesitation. Plenty of us would kiss and greet when both parties were naked, or mid-bathing suit change. In the States, teammates do get changed near one another or in open dressing areas, and are methodical about not being fully naked around one another. They most definitely would never kiss, hug or greet another teammate at a moment that they were in the nude.

After the workout, or really after any workout in any gym I encountered, the showers were open. Women of all shape and sizes shower naked, of course. They talk, they shampoo, they shave, and they take their time.

I have since worked at ten gyms in the U.S., and at every single one I am confident in saying that such openness and liberalness of the body does not happen. All showers in our gyms are partitioned off and are private, and if they are not, people tend to shower in their bathing suit. Women do not even walk from the shower to their locker nude, some change their clothes in the shower stall, and some bundle up with their towels and cover as much skin as possible so that others do not see or judge them.

It all comes back to judgment. *The minute we stop judging ourselves and allowing ourselves to be judged, we will experience freedom.*

The French take on the human body is one of the healthiest and most liberating that I have ever experienced. I challenge you to start getting naked more often and see what it does for you.

Since you are going to be nude more frequently, it's time you start looking at yourself with new, kind eyes. What little pleasures do you get from looking at yourself naked? I ask the question in a non-sexual way; what are the things about your body that bring a smile of appreciation and thankfulness to your face? Corporeal appreciation can derive from the smallest detail to the most obvious asset. What *petites* parts of your body bring you *plaisir*? Do you like the freckles on your kneecaps, the whiteness of your smile, your crooked snaggle-tooth, your pronounced dimples, your uniquely awkward ear lobes, or perhaps your natural beauty marks?

Is it hard or easy for you to come up with your list? If it was hard, you are not alone. Some of us don't yet know ourselves, both physically and emotionally. Yes, we also are afraid to really take a look at ourselves fully naked. We are afraid to truly strip down, both physically and emotionally, and to have nothing to hide behind.

When battling this process of discovery, many of us get sidetracked by self-sabotage. Everyone's form of self-sabotage is different, but we engage in such behavior for the same fundamental reasons: we are afraid that when we get fully naked, physically and metaphorically, that we will have nothing to really offer. So instead of allowing ourselves to really see ourselves, we feel safer sabotaging our own efforts so that we have an excuse to blame for our lives gone wrong.

For some of us, food is the ultimate weapon of self-destruction that prevents us from approaching the Bridge. My disordered relationship with food prevented me for years from really taking the first real step into the unknown. It was much safer to wish away my insecurities and to hide behind the mask of food, which served as an excuse not to grow. I was convinced that I was going to finally be happy after I lost those "last five pounds." Others hide behind designer clothes and expensive cars. They never leave the house without makeup on or never admit to buying clothes at Target or Wal-Mart. Out to impress others, we fool ourselves into believing we are something we are not. When we lose ourselves in creating a materialistic, class-based identity, our developmental selves drown and are forgotten.

Each person's shield of protection is different, but in the end, we are all doing the same thing. We are avoiding having to work through the wounds of our past or having to discover how such a past has molded us into the complexly beautiful individual we are today. If we never let our guard down, we will never have the opportunity to embrace ourselves for who we really are. We will never love our skin and will never share what we are meant to with others.

So, get naked. Can you spend ten minutes naked in a room by yourself? This challenge is not for the light of heart. Be comforted in knowing that the average person is most insecure when fully unclothed. If you really want to break free of body image insecurity, commit yourself to loving yourself naked. Once your overly critical eyes begin to see that *you* look good naked, it will bring you freedom in every other aspect of living.

Too many of us are not comfortable naked. Some of the most confident women I have ever met confess to me that they cower from themselves when naked in a mirror. These women also have sex only with the lights off, all the while wishing they were wilder and more adventurous in their skin. Let's face it, we are all terrified of rejection. We all examine our bodies and wonder if our parts look like they're supposed to. Should we shave our bikini area, get a Brazilian, or let ourselves be natural? How do our breasts compare? Are our butts too big or too small?

Try to imagine yourself in a world where a body is never rejected and where all bodies are considered beautiful. That world is France, and it does exist. Just knowing that that world exists can help you realize that your body, flaws and all, is too beautiful to ever be rejected.

Needing the same push myself, I decided to start sleeping naked. The first night I did, I didn't want to. I was comfortably bundled up in my oversized t-shirt and plaid pajama pants, and had eaten too much at dinner and so was uncomfortably bloated. Being naked while feeling like your stomach is poking out an extra eight inches is not what I consider appealing or encouraging for a non-nudist. The truth is that good change is uncomfortable. You have to allow yourself to step outside of the box of the familiar and push yourself to doing what is so uncomfortably different.

My first night naked was bliss. I was more aware of the smoothness of my skin, the tautness of my body and the movement of my limbs throughout the night. The psychological freedom was almost as enthralling as unwrapping a new present on Christmas morning. Just one night of nakedness, a full ten-hour slumber, was like re-gifting my body back to myself.

Night two was deeper sleep than I've had in months. Usually doomed to waking up in fits of sweat and restlessness, I slept peacefully straight through the night. Waking up to yourself naked in the morning is one of the first steps to starting your day in appreciation of your body.

The third night into my experiment, I had had an overwhelming day at work. Too exhausted to take my clothes off, I plopped into bed and passed out without a second thought as to what I was wearing. Subsequently, I had a restless night of sleep and woke up feeling anxious and rushed in the morning. Was it because I didn't sleep naked? No, of course not; I do, however, attribute the difference to my negligence in properly lulling my mind and body before turning in for the night. I took my American day and turned it into an American night.

What I want us to understand is that a few moments of silence, peacefulness and rest will bode for nights of better rest, mornings of a more innate confidence, and a generally slower pace of life. Even if the slower pace of life only exists in our minds, our bodies will follow suit and stay healthier.

The truth is that in order to make our lives easier, we often first have to make them harder. We have to consciously choose to do something different, stop doing something we are accustomed to, or start doing something we've never tried before. *Change is often uncomfortable, because we are letting go of the familiar.* Even fear can be comfortable, because it is often so familiar. Letting go of our fears and our habits can be as painful as ripping off a band-aid; it is a temporary, yet necessary pain of the healing process.

CHOOSING TO COURT YOURSELF

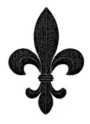

Another shaky board on the bridge that trips up courageous crossers is meekness. Meekness, or being overly submissive and compliant, is a good quality is some aspects of life, but in the development of self, it can be disabling.

How well do you receive compliments? How well do you accept gifts and praise from others? The confident journeyer relishes in such delight, for they know themselves and they know their worth. Do not be meek in accepting compliments from others. When complimented, thank the person and remember that their compliment should uplift you, but not define you.

Are you one of those people who minimize and deflect praise? You feel that anyone being so nice to you must be insincere or trying to use you for something. You are aware of an innate mistrust of the people around you. What you may not be aware of is that you have more mistrust with yourself than with others. You are more of a stranger to yourself than the street passerby who compliments you on your sweater.

I have a girlfriend who has bounced around unhealthy relationships for years, always going back to the same type of guy that tends to be negligent and emotionally detached. She berates herself for drifting toward the same prototype and is puzzled at her undeniable attraction to Mr. Wrong. When a good guy does come her way, she panics at the attention and consideration he gives her and feels that she is undeserving of such positive attention. Attentiveness makes her feel uncomfortable, unsettled almost, for she feels that her past proves that she deserves nothing of the sort of man who makes her feel safe, cherished, and sexy.

To my friend, this is fundamentally not a dating issue. No, beneath the thickness of her emotional skin lies a tender naivety and fear of self-discovery. She says that she loves her body, but she is a perfectionist in the process of accepting her skin. She obsesses about her daily workouts, skin cleansers, and invests religiously in Clinique and plastic surgery. She loves her skin when she feels beautiful externally. She has no concept however of the depth of her beauty beneath the skin. She is afraid to let herself be properly loved because she still holds on to the pain and insecurities of past relationships and betrayals. It is as if she has stunted her own emotional growth. My friend will never experience positive bliss in her orbit until she comes to accept herself. Once she accepts herself and lets go of the painful memories of her past, she will begin to see the beauty in her heart. It is not until she has a mastered understanding of her own glorious femininity that she will truly arrive at the point in which she can live with a *skinny, sexy mind.*

Love your body. It is not until you arrive at a moment of total body acceptance that you can begin to fully live and love your life.

As I have pointed out, loving your body is beyond the physical. You need to understand *yourself* before you can love and appreciate the peaks and crevices of your body.

Think about your body as a living art sculpture. Every day, you are shaping and perfecting it in some way. Either through spiritual enlightenment, emotional growth, or physical training, you are chipping away the stone and coming to life. You are the Michelangelo of yourself. You were made beautiful; it is up to you to recognize and embrace your individual beauty. Once you love yourself for your unique beauty and personality, then the Michelangelo in you will begin to shine through. Your confidence and *joie* will magnetize others your way and people will begin to see you through rose-colored glasses. When someone loves their body, they love their life and it is obvious. This is the making of a *skinny, sexy mind*.

THE JOURNEY OF CHOICE
Skinny, Sexy *à la carte*
Qui ne risque rien n'a rien.
[Nothing ventured, nothing gained.]

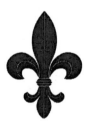

i. Skinny, Sexy SUMMARY:

The power of development lies entirely in our minds and is dependent on what thoughts we choose to think. We are what we think, and we ultimately have the power of choice in every thought we think.

ii. Skinny, Sexy REFLECTION:

What are your glaring stains of your personal past and how do they influence the way you live?

Do you allow yourself to be a victim to these past experiences or are you thankful for the ways in which they have changed your life?

iii. Skinny, Sexy PERSONAL APPLICATION:

Practice repeating the phrase *"I am strong and I am beautiful"* to yourself ten times a day for the next week and make note of how much it impacts you internally. Remember, the body listens to what the mind thinks!

iv. Skinny, Sexy EATING:

Change is often uncomfortable, because we are letting go of the familiar. Make a commitment to let go of the familiar in your food preferences. Be open minded to try out new foods, new ways of cooking, and new ways of thinking about your relationship with food in your life. Try to eat one new thing and to cook one new recipe weekly.

v. Skinny, Sexy YOU

Nothing draws admiration more than authenticity. Be strong and un-apologetically authentic in who you are, and when you do, you will have no regrets in life. Nothing is more authentic than you naked. Try the naked exercise that is explained in this chapter and start committing to loving and accepting yourself at your most vulner-able state.

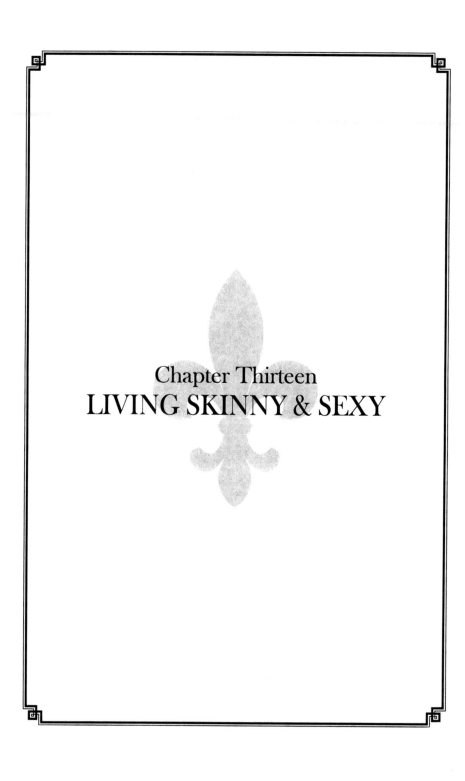

Chapter Thirteen
LIVING SKINNY & SEXY

Chapter Thirteen
LIVING SKINNY & SEXY

French people master *joie de vivre* because they have learned that life comes alive when the little things in it are appreciated. One of the most pivotal examples of appreciation that I admired in my French friends was their ability appreciate *themselves*. Not once do I recall a Frenchman apologizing to me for who he was, what he was like, or for his quirks. Similar to the way in which the French understand how to discover the complexities and tannins in vintage wines, they have developed a powerful ability to savor the unique, human complexities of their own beauty.

During training sessions with clients, I emphasize the mantra that the body achieves what the mind believes. Ninety percent of any success in sculpting the body and reshaping a lifestyle is dependent on a person's thought-life. Like my French friends, my clients' appreciation of self gives them the seed for healthy thought patterns, resulting in an uncanny ability to live a lifestyle of balance and health.

The mind is a powerful thing and the thoughts that you allow it to dwell on will have a significant impact upon your life, your own self-perception, and on the way others perceive you. Your ability to live freely and confidently in your own body will only derive from a mind that is focused on living life to the fullest and is free from being focused on achieving a perfect body. Life should be about living, not about achieving.

I was once in a room with thirty beautiful women for a party. It was a girls' night out kind of party, women aged between 23 and 57, all in the prime of their lives and beauty. These were not your average looking girls, but women that would turn your head in the street. Everyone was dressed nicely, stylishly even, and hair and makeup was meticulously done on all.

Yet, looking around at the room, there was an absolute lack of self-confidence and presence missing. The uncertainty that permeated the room highlighted the two issues that plague women and emanate insecurity. The first is that women, when surrounded by other women, can be easily intimidated by one another. Subsequently, they compare themselves and end up feeling even more insecurely jealous. The other thing I noticed was how none of these women seemed confident in knowing themselves, which is another pitfall along the pathway for those pursuing a *skinny, sexy mind.*

Comparing oneself to others is one of the most treacherous and tragic practices of our society. And it's no wonder that we love to compare, because we are taught that game from our earliest youth. We are surrounded by cultural reminders at every turn and we buy into a culture that praises those who are the most stylish, in shape, successful and beautiful. We do it to ourselves. We do it in athletics, academics, the arts, and in our social circles. To a certain extent, competitiveness can be healthy and can refine us as individuals. Taken to an extreme, it can destroy that which we know of ourselves, causing us to live in a perpetual cycle of dissatisfaction.

This is where the French women set themselves apart. Comparing yourself to others will always ultimately end with making you feel shoddy. French women embrace their uniqueness, their personal poise, and their inner-most selves. In fact, the "inner circle" of a French woman is so private, so privileged, and so safe, that she is free to truly know and embrace herself. The French are very selective about who is granted entrance into their inner circle of trust. Sociologists concur that the French tend to focus on the quality of friendships versus the quantity of friends that they have. Americans, on the other hand, like to maximize their networking possibilities and social status by having as many friends as possible. Encouraged by the self-empowerment of her inner circle, the French woman is undeterred by the average passer-by on the street, indifferent to others' opinions of her, and carries herself with glamour and poise because, well, it makes *her* happy. *In other words, her beauty is for herself.*

In my example of the thirty beautiful women, please remember that everyone was dressed up, bottles of good wine were being passed around freely and joyfully, and smiles were on every face. However, in only five out of thirty women, did I see women who I could tell *knew* they were beautiful. They weren't arrogant and they weren't over-confident. They weren't the skinniest or even the prettiest by cultural standards. They *were* the most beautiful though; they were sexy. It was written on their faces, in the confident way in which they walked, and in their eyes – it was clear to the passerby that they *knew* themselves and were at peace in their own skin. They weren't ashamed of their quirks, their uniqueness, their blemishes, or their extra ten pounds. They loved themselves and every curve of their bodies. It was beautiful to behold.

That is where the French excel; the French practically worship the human form. French love skin and flesh. They admire beauty in a woman's body, in its curves, and in its uniqueness, because they understand that beauty comes in all shapes and sizes. No matter the shape or size, beauty captivates. America is obsessed with perfection. France sees beauty in all forms.

French women are sexy. French women believe that they are sexy. Sexy is a state of mind. And remember, the mind is a powerful thing.

American women are beautiful. "Sexy," though, is a word reserved for the likes of MTV, *Cosmopolitan,* celebrity lists, and Brad Pitt. Most American women wouldn't dare use the adjective sexy for themselves. Justin Timberlake is bringing sexy back, not us. We are more familiar with the words "diet," "surgery," "gym," "cellulite" and "jiggle." We are even afraid of what the word sexy means. Does it mean throwing aside modest values and embracing casual sex? Does it mean exposing our nipples publicly Janet Jackson style or taking a pole-dancing class? Does it mean we have to be pursuing men or seeking attention? No, no, no and no.

Sexy, simply put, is a healthy self-image. Sexy is rejecting the temptation to compare our bodies to the women beside us. Sexy is refusing to continue to prescribe to our own mantras of body dysmorphia and self-loathing. Sexy is loving ourselves for what is *below* the skin. Sexiness is knowing your true self and living life from the heart. Sexy is the beauty that shines from the eyes and draws others to its warmth.

Our over-critical nature and society prevents our minds from having the freedom to accept our own individual beauty. There is no excuse, though; blaming it on society is just a cop-out. We learned earlier that everything in life is mental and we have control over our minds. If your mind hears enough times that you are sexy, your body will start to believe it.

French women know they are beautiful, they know their beauty. Knowledge is power, and in this case, the knowledge of beauty empowers them to be sexy. American women want to be beautiful. We typically don't know if we are or not; we yearn to be told it by others. As little girls we dream of being Sleeping Beauty, we are fixated by the Miss America Pageant, and we believe that we will grow up to look like our beloved Barbie doll. Our world of childhood innocence is shattered upon arrival in adolescence, when we realize that we are flawed compared to the retouched images we so admired as children. Here begins the destruction of our fragile body image.

Every American woman needs to embark on a personal path of self-reflection. Such a journey will provide countless personal discoveries and will ultimately result in the ability to not only believe in your beauty and joy for life, but to *own* it.

Here is a challenge to begin your self-reflection: make a list of 365 reasons why you are uniquely beautiful and why you love yourself. Write it out and then type it up. It will change your vision of yourself, I promise. Anticipate that this challenge will take you more than one sitting. Mine took four months. When you are finished you will see yourself with new eyes. You will not only know your beauty, but you will arrive at the point where you actually appreciate yourself and embrace yourself, flaws and all. You will believe wholeheartedly that you are distinctively sexy.

The following is a list that will help inspire you to new levels of self-appreciation.

SEXY WAYS TO APPRECIATE YOU

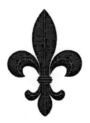

- When it rains, go stand in it and smile. You will remember what it feels like to be a child.

- Make your bed, naked.

- Do your laundry in sexy heels.

- Repeat: "Self-esteem is not a dress size; it is a state of mind."

- Sit up straight when driving.

- Celebrate small victories in your life as if they were huge.

- Improve your posture; stand with your chest out, shoulders back.

- Be proud of who you are and of what makes you tick; make it show.

- Happiness doesn't start five pounds from now; happiness starts *today*.

- Detail the interior of your car: you will feel like you are driving in pure luxury.

- Lather yourself in lotion when you dry off from a shower. Caressing every inch of your skin will lend your mind to think kinder thoughts about every centimeter of your body.

- Take pride in pampering yourself.

- Experiment weekly with different cooking styles, spices, and seasonings.

- Figure out exactly what moves your heart, and pursue that single thing.

- Shave your legs for yourself.

- Educate yourself daily on something that peaks your interest.

- When drinking wine, allow the wine to linger upon the back of your tongue.

- Find positive adjectives to associate with each one of your so-called problem areas.

- Sleep nude without pajamas or buy a new piece of sexy lingerie for yourself.

- Wear a fun hairstyle with confidence.

- Stay in on a Saturday night and have a movie-marathon of your favorite films. You will feel like you had a relaxing, luxurious weekend away and will feel especially refreshed for the coming week.

- Wear a thong (and nothing else) around the house as if it's a natural thing to do.

- Snuggle yourself up in a large down comforter and read a book.

- Walk confidently, with your head held high and shoulders back, and notice the attention you will get.

- Find a local wine festival; go and educate yourself on diversifying your taste palate.

- Take a candlelit bath, and sip your favorite beverage (wine, tea, hot chocolate); a book or a DVD playing on your laptop will amplify the relaxation.

- Go to a matinee at the local theatre by yourself on a weekday.

- Spoil yourself and get your nails done.

- Keep a dictionary in your bathroom – learn a new vocabulary word daily while brushing your teeth and use it in a sentence that day. You will feel smart and sexy as you stimulate your mind intellectually.

- Dance around naked when you are getting dressed.

- Take a yoga class and learn to appreciate the movement of your body.

- Learn how to lift from a certified personal trainer or a friend familiar with fitness and feel your body being sculpted; as you build strength you will feel internally strong and sexy too.

- Personalize your license plate to something uniquely you.

- If you feel frumpy, be sure to wear a matching pair of bra and panties. It will lift your mood and opinion of self.

- Spend ten minutes a day stretching and elongating your limbs; as you become more and more limber you will have a greater awareness of your body and muscles and subsequently a greater appreciation for the unique wonder that is your body.

- Save all of your change and create a discretionary fund – when you save enough, treat yourself to a professional massage.

- When you walk into work for the day, exclaim confidently to yourself... "I am sexy. I am smart. I am strong."

LIVING SKINNY & SEXY
Skinny, Sexy *à la carte*
Quand on veut, on peut.
[When there's a will, there's a way.]

i. Skinny, Sexy SUMMARY:

The French master *joie de vivre* because they have learned that life comes alive when the little things in it are appreciated; moreover, *joie de vivre* includes the appreciation of one's own self.

ii. Skinny, Sexy REFLECTION:

Do you know that you are beautiful? *What are your qualities inside and out that make you beautiful?*

iii. Skinny, Sexy PERSONAL APPLICATION:

The mind is a powerful thing and the thoughts that you allow it to dwell on will have a significant impact upon your life, your own self-perception, and on the way others perceive you. Life should be about living, not about achieving. What areas of your life are you obsessed about achieving? What do you need to do to flip that mentality from a focus on achievement to a focus on living and *experiencing?*

Start your list of 365 reasons why you are beautiful and why you love yourself. This will take a long time, commit to completing the list. It will be a transforming and enlightening experience.

iv. Skinny, Sexy EATING:

Identify three foods that make you feel sexy and good from the inside out.

v. Skinny, Sexy YOU:

Make a plan of action to incorporate regular moments of self-reflection and self-analysis into your life. Self-reflection enables you to not only know the power of your beauty and purpose, but to *own* it.

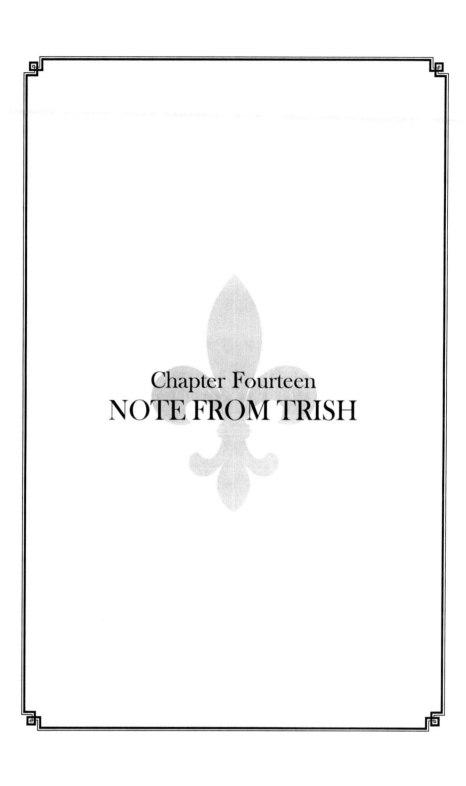

Chapter Fourteen
NOTE FROM TRISH

Chapter Fourteen
NOTE FROM TRISH

Thank you for sharing in my journey as you read this book. I hope that you are on the path to loving the skin you are in and embracing *joie de vivre* in your life. Please let me know how this book has changed the way you think about yourself and love yourself. A community of confidence is built through sharing experiences and I would love to hear about yours.

Be strong. Be confident, and, most importantly, be you.

Connect with me and share your thoughts:

trish@trishblackwell.com

Appendix I
LIVING NUTRITIONALLY
100 RULES TO LIVE AND EAT BY

Appendix I
LIVING NUTRITIONALLY
100 RULES TO LIVE AND EAT BY

1. Breakfast is a must.

2. Prescribe to the 3-HOUR RULE. Eat something small at least every three hours no matter what; it will help keep your metabolism high and active.

3. Remember: you are what you eat. Eat nutritiously and splurge moderately to achieve a balanced diet. If you eat healthy food, you will feel healthy on the inside.

4. Do not obsess about food. Obsessing about food only puts you under the control of food, and food should never have that much power in your life.

5. Make water your drink of choice. Always carry a bottle with you.

6. Drink cold water (less than 72 degrees). It takes your body 25 calories to warm it up; drinking 1 liter/day equals losing 5 pounds/ year.

7.   Add water to fruit juice. Fruit juice is high in calories and sugars, and adding water will cut down on your calorie consumption.

8.   Blot pizza and other fatty foods with a napkin. Doing so can save you one tsp/week of fat, equaling one cup of fat/year. It is OK to have food like this on occasion, as long as it is in moderation.

9.   Take a calcium supplement. 1,800mg of calcium/day can block absorption of up to 80 calories of your daily intake. This will also improve your bone density for stronger and healthier bones.

10.   Eat without doing anything else. Sit down at a table and really enjoy what you are eating and tasting.

11.   Drink a sip of water between every three bites of food when eating.

12.   Chew a strongly flavored gum while cooking to ward off the temptation to pick.

13.   Get into the habit of making hot organic herbal tea at night to ward off snack cravings and help put you in your Zen.

14.   Drink 10 ounces of water before you eat anything. It will give you more sensory awareness of your fullness while you eat and help with digestion.

15.   Eat high fiber food with every meal. Aim for 30g of fiber daily. You will feel full and satisfied longer and will have a healthier gastrointestinal system.

16.   Shop locally and eat what's in season. If an item doesn't have a season, you should limit the amount you eat of it.

17. Steam fresh veggies for no longer than two minutes in order to retain the most nutrients possible. You will know they are perfectly done when they turn a vibrant color. Overcooking vegetables will make them lose much of their nutritional value.

18. Real food can never be overrated. Processed foods have a time and place for convenience, but contain unhealthy amounts of sodium and additives needed for preservation.

19. Keep sodium intake to 1500mg/day. This is much lower than the Recommended Daily Allotment (RDA) of 2,400mg and will prevent water retention and bloating. Never add salt to food. Never.

20. Instead of salt, use fresh cilantro and fresh basil: grind them up together and use garlic powder and onion powder to season fresh salmon and boneless, skinless chicken.

21. Drink 3/4 of your body weight in ounces of water every day. For example, if you weigh 160lbs, then you should drink 120 ounces of water. It will increase your metabolism and help you differentiate properly between thirst and hunger pangs.

22. Allow yourself one cheat meal and cheat drink per week.

23. Never do mixed drinks with high calorie mixers. Always choose diet or no-calorie mixers; alcohol has enough calories and sugars to make the drink a splurge for the nutrition-conscious consumer.

24. Prepare Monday through Friday's food on Sunday so that you have no excuse to eat out or visit the vending machine at the office. Use plastic Tupperware containers so that all you need to do in the morning is grab and go. Packing your food for the day should take less than ten minutes. You will save calories and tons of money.

25. Never eat pre-prepared tuna salad, chicken salad or pasta salad from the grocery store or a restaurant. "Salad" may make you feel like you're making a healthy choice, but typically these "salads" are loaded with fat-filled mayo that skyrockets you above the recommended daily allowance (RDA) of 64g fat/day.

26. Make homemade chicken salad with low-fat yogurt or Greek yogurt instead of full fat mayonnaise.

27. Have a stash of protein snacks for nights when you have cravings: endamame beans, almonds, cottage cheese, whey protein shakes, and yogurt. You will feel satisfied from indulging and your waistline will never know the difference.

28. Write down everything you eat, and be aware of exactly what you put into your body. Dieters who keep a food journal lose twice as much weight.

29. Multi-vitamin supplements can help increase your body's natural metabolic rate when taken regularly: make it a daily habit.

30. Take Viactin multivitamins or chocolate flavored calcium chews. If you save them for lunch, you will avoid a mid-afternoon chocolate fix.

31. Make afternoon coffee a habit. Mid-afternoon caffeine will stimulate your metabolism and energy. If you don't like coffee, treat yourself to a sugar free hot chocolate.

32. Plug your ears if you hear about a new crash-diet or magic weight-loss pill. If it sounds too good to be true, it is.

33. Stop comparing your body and your diet to other people's; it will only bring negativity upon the way you approach food and

accept your body how it is. Remember, everybody is different and you have to <u>know</u> your body and what works for you!

34.   Never eat less than 1200 calories/day. Doing so puts your body into starvation mode, where it becomes a fat-storage machine.

35.   Make it a post-grocery store routine to divvy out portions of snacks, cereal, etc. and put them into zip-lock baggies for easy convenience later.

36.   Look up restaurant nutrition facts online and memorize three healthy options for the restaurants you frequent the most.

37.   When buying a lunch, snack, or dinner out, pay cash. People who pay cash typically spend 30% less per meal than those who use a debit or credit card. This will lower your calorie-intake, as well.

38.   An apple a day keeps the doctor away. Sometimes old wives tales are full of truth. The pectin in an apple helps to cleanse the digestive system and is considered to help prevent some forms of cancer.

39.   Ask for half of your meal to be boxed at a restaurant before it is served to you. The waiter will bring the second half out when they bring you your bill.

40.   Allow food to touch every part of the inside of your mouth: feel the difference of texture and taste upon the roof of your mouth versus your tongue, and experiment with feeling the fullness of the food's taste by allowing it to linger on different parts of your tongue as you chew.

41.   Never allow yourself to say you are on a diet. A diet has a beginning and an end (*die*-t), and you will set yourself up for failure.

42. Make healthy eating a *lifestyle*.

43. Never eat a meal without some form of protein.

44. Eat carbohydrates early in the day, and avoid them like the plague at night.

45. Pre-exercise, eat carbohydrates for energy. Post-exercise, eat protein to enable muscle recovery and the development of your lean muscle mass (and your metabolism).

46. Help boost your metabolism by taking 1000 mcg of Chromium Picolinate daily. Chromium helps regulate your body's natural blood sugar levels and helps the body to break down carbohydrates.

47. Sleep 8 hours a night. Sleeping burns calories and a well-rested body has a naturally higher metabolism. Sleeping produces a chemical mix of hormones released by the body, including leptin and a natural form of human growth hormone (HGH). Leptin helps control appetite, and HGH stimulates metabolism and natural muscle development. Lack of sleep increases cortisol, a stress hormone, in the body. High levels of cortisol promote fat storage and fatigue.

48. Eat as many vegetables as your heart desires. You will feel full and decrease desire for other food.

49. Food that comes through your car window is not food. Enough said.

50. Never skip a meal.

51. Bring a platter of fresh fruit, veggies, and fat-free dip to food-oriented activities. An all-you-can-eat social buffet can be a dangerous pitfall, and having healthy options will enable you to munch without feeling socially awkward.

52. Eat to live - don't live to eat.

53. You can never sneak food by your body. Your body never lies, and the unhealthy things you put into your body will eventually show. Treat your body with respect.

54. Add herbs to foods like vegetables and chicken; flavors will be intensified and you will find healthy food more exciting.

55. Hot spices and cayenne pepper added to food will help increase your metabolism while you eat.

56. Calculate your Basal Metabolic Rate. This will tell you how many calories your body burns while resting. **Women**: BMR = 655 + (4.35 x weight in pounds) + (4.7 x height in inches) - (4.7 x age in years). **Men**: BMR = 66 + (6.23 x weight in pounds) + (12.7 x height in inches) - (6.8 x age in years).

57. Know how to ballpark how many calories you actually need daily to be healthy. Multiply your BMR according to the following appropriate categories: 1.2 (sedentary), 1.375 (workout moderately 2-3x/week), 1.55 (workout moderately 3-5x/week), and 1.725 (workout intensely 6-7x/week).

58. Eating a form of whey (milk-based) protein before going to bed will increase your metabolism while you sleep. Low-fat cottage cheese takes four hours or more for your body to break down, so your first four hours of sleep are extra calorie burning!

59. Buy only the fruits and vegetables that are in season and buy them as often as possible from local Farmer's Markets or in the organic section of your grocery store. This will ensure that you are not consuming pesticides and that what you are eating is full of nutrition. You will also find that what you are eating will taste richer and be more vibrant in flavor.

60.   Pre-planning a nighttime snack will help you control unhealthy nighttime eating. People tend to crave what they anticipate; if you anticipate and plan on eating something healthy at night, you will actually crave it.

61.   Obesity is contagious. Unhealthy eating among friends usually spurs more unhealthy eating. Make a pact between friends to encourage one another to make nutritious choices.

62.   Green tea is a natural thermogenic. Supplement with 270mg/day or three cups of green tea to help increase the rate at which your body burns calories.

63.   Eat healthy Omega-3 fats like extra virgin olive oil and walnuts; your body needs a certain amount of healthy fat to function at its highest levels of efficiency.

64.   Brush and floss your teeth between meals; clean teeth and a fresh mouth will minimize your desire to snack unnecessarily.

65.   Oatmeal is the perfect high-energy breakfast choice. Healthy, low glycemic-index carbs deliver long-lasting energy and a metabolic boost in the morning.

66.   Choose egg whites for a fat-burning breakfast: be creative with presentation. Egg whites are delicious in low-free cottage cheese, with mango-peach salsa, and scrambled with low-fat mozzarella cheese, just to name a few possibilities.

67.   Educate yourself. Be a label reader.

68.   Know what true serving sizes are in order to appropriately control your food portions.

69.   For a balanced meal, divide your plate into quarters: fill ¼ of

the plate with carbohydrates, ¼ of the plate with a lean protein, and ½ of the plate with vegetables.

70. Never teach your children that they must finish everything on their plate.

71. Encourage yourself and your children to listen to your bodies, eat until you are satisfied, not until you are full. If you eat until you are full, you will probably have eaten too much.

72. Limit daily sugar intake to 125g.

73. Keep blood sugar in check (and thereby avoid energy crashes and food cravings) by avoiding food with added sugars.

74. Eating "fake" sugars are just as destructive to your body as regular sugar. Anything that is chemically manufactured to substitute sugar for fewer calories will result in adverse affects on your body. Your body still recognizes it as sugar, but it is overloaded with unnatural chemicals that throw off your body's natural pH balance and will cause your sweet tooth to increase.

75. The body is dependent upon a balanced internal pH for optimal health. Eat more alkalinizing foods than acidifying foods in your diet. Alkalinizing foods include sprouts, fruit, vegetables, nuts and live grains. Acidifying foods include meat, dairy, caffeine, alcohol and anything overly processed.

76. Your diet should consist of 70% alkalinizing foods and 30% acidifying foods. You will be amazed at your improved state of health and increased energy levels if you follow these guidelines.

77. When eating carbohydrates, always choose complex ones. To remember what complex carbohydrates are, remember

that brown and dark carbohydrates always win over white. For example, sweet potatoes are a better choice than baked potatoes and brown rice is healthier than white rice. Whole grain, complex carbohydrates reduce plunges in blood sugar levels and are more effectively processed by the body for energy rather than storage.

78. Know your diet pitfalls. Generate a plan of action to avoid falling into unhealthy eating.

79. Forgive yourself for overeating binges. Feeling guilty, angry, or depressed only continues the overeating cycle and permits the calorie overload.

80. Incorporate flaxseed oil into your diet. Flaxseed lowers cholesterol and susceptibility to coronary heart disease, is high in soluble fiber, and is considered to lower cancer risk.

81. Load up on vitamin Bs, found in many protein sources – they will rev up your metabolism and overall mood.

82. Clean out your cupboards and fridge; declare your household a healthy food only house. Never buy foods that you can't resist or problematic goodies.

83. Listen to your hunger: fuel your body when your body tells you. First make sure you actually are hungry and aren't just bored or thirsty.

84. Find distractions for yourself if you are bored; do not give in to boredom eating because it becomes mindless and you end up consuming up to five times more than you initially intended.

85. Every time you consider eating something, evaluate whether or not it is going to fuel your body towards health or towards deterioration.

86. Food should never be a reward. Yes, it should be enjoyed with pleasure, but avoid associating it as a reward; those who consider it a reward tend to overeat at night or when stressed as a subconscious reward after a long day.

87. To combat sugar cravings, visualize the sugar and fat in the food you crave and visualize it adding an inch to your waistline. The body stores unnecessary calories and it is typically in the places we least want it to.

88. When grocery shopping, shop the perimeter of the store; always buy what is fresh and in season. Perimeter shopping will help you avoid aisles that are filled with processed, sugary, and generally nutrient-void food choices.

89. Enjoy an occasional glass of red wine. The antioxidants in red wine will help fight damaging free radicals at the molecular level in your body.

90. Do not be obsessive about weighing yourself; body weight can fluctuate to 8 pounds depending on water retention and menstrual cycles. Often, those who get easily discouraged by weigh-ins are more prone to indulge in sweets to console themselves.

91. Eat carbohydrates pre-workout and first thing in the morning; your body will burn them off immediately and they will give you a tremendous amount of energy.

92. Consider supplementing your workouts with glutamine. Glutamine will help your muscles recover more quickly and will maximize the lean muscle building benefits of your workout. Remember, the more lean muscle mass you have, the higher you metabolism will be. Take 5-15g/day as a supplement daily.

93.   Choose a food accountability partner: a friend, husband, trainer, or neighbor who can help encourage your healthy eating lifestyle and with whom you can share creative new recipes and ideas.

94.   Your drinks also count as calories – make sure you include them in your calorie awareness and chose them wisely.

95.   Know that there are 3,200 calories in one pound of fat. Every calorie you take in matters!

96.   Eat within the first 30 minutes of waking up; this will rev up your metabolism. If you delay or skip breakfast, you are sabotaging your metabolism and setting yourself up to burn calories at a slower rate.

97.   Grocery shop with a list. This keeps you focused on the necessities and you will be much less likely to veer towards the snack isle.

98.   Keep a box of protein bars, nuts and bottled water in your car trunk so that you are always prepared with a snack and have no excuse for skipping meals or going to a drive-thru.

99.   Remember: under-eating and skipping meals will only put you into a catabolic state where your body eats away your precious lean muscle and stores fat.

100. Make lunch a larger meal than dinner; over-loading on calories at night and skimping on calories throughout the day leads to storage of body fat. When the body has unneeded calories, it stores them.

LIVING NUTRITIONALLY
Skinny, Sexy *à la carte*
Il faut manger pour vivre, et non pas vivre pour manger.
[Eat to live, don't live to eat.]

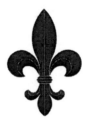

i. Skinny, Sexy SUMMARY:

Healthy and balanced eating is grounded in choosing natural, un-processed, balanced foods and in listening to one's body's needs.

ii. Skinny, Sexy REFLECTION:

Does the food you eat make you feel good, or does it make you feel bloated and/or cranky? *Food should always make you feel better.* How often do you feel hungry, and do you listen to your hunger when your body is speaking to you? *Hunger is a sign of a high metabolism and a sure sign to eat.* Do you feel energized and alive after eating or weighed down and heavy? *Food should always make you feel light and energized.* If you don't feel that way, it is likely that you are over-eating.

iii. Skinny, Sexy PERSONAL APPLICATION:

Tackle committing to five new nutritional goals from this chapter's list per week until you have mastered them all. Be patient with yourself and applaud yourself for every positive change you make in regards to your relationship with food. Remember, these are life changes – take your time and commit to a healthy mind and healthy body.

iv. Skinny, Sexy EATING:

Here you have it, your 100 nutritional rules to live by!

v. Skinny, Sexy YOU:

Treat your body with respect, listen to its needs, and nourish your body as it needs to be nourished in order to sustain your celebratory state of living.

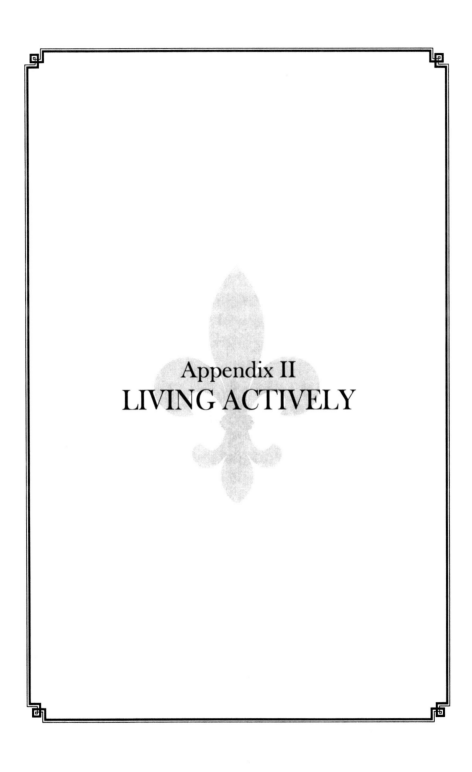

Appendix II
LIVING ACTIVELY

Appendix II
LIVING ACTIVELY

THE FRENCH WORKOUT:

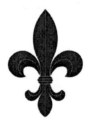

- Walk everywhere you go.

- Always take the stairs, always.

- Move your car as little as possible.

- Bicycle to work.

- Gasoline is expensive – use it as little as possible.

- Use your lunch hour to walk to the farthest café in town, meet a friend there, and then walk back.

- Enjoy the variance of life – change up your activities on a daily basis.

- Join a gym, but don't go there every day; make sure you exercise outside.

- If you like to go out at night, go somewhere you can dance and move.

- Grocery shop on a daily basis – it will make you walk around more and your food will always be fresh.

- Take walks with friends.

- Get a dog and exercise with it.

- Hike with your family on weekends.

- Sit up straight all day; it will keep your core and abs more active and toned.

- Practice perfect posture: it will make you look thinner and more confident.

- Make the intention of your exercise for your health rather than for the number on the scale.

- Exercise isn't necessarily about getting sweaty and dirty, but about moving your body and feeling alive.

- Cycling is a great way to see the countryside and tone your legs at the same time.

- Exercise is meant to be social: get involved in a local run or bike group or meet others at a gym through group exercise classes. The more camaraderie and accountability you experience with exercise, the more you will succeed and enjoy yourself.

- Dance.

- Weekend afternoons are meant to be spent outside either walking around town shopping, walking trails with your family, or playing tennis.

- Move your body: do what you enjoy doing and you will be more likely to stay committed to it over your lifetime.

- Stretch for two minutes every few hours throughout the day. You will find that it will increase the blood flow to your body giving you more energy, attentiveness and ability to manage stress.

- Take three breaks every day to breathe. On your breathing break, take three deep breaths, inhale deeply and exhale slowly and fully. The breath will infuse you with life and energy.

LIVING ACTIVELY IN AMERICA:

- Cardio isn't just about keeping your weight down; it's about heart health.

- If you struggle to do cardio, do it first thing in the morning so it becomes a habit and you aren't tempted to skip it at the end of the day.

- Commit to be fit – find a workout buddy who will help keep your motivation up when you are getting discouraged and you will be able to do the same for them.

- Commit to a purpose – sign up for a local race or event so that you have a purpose to stay committed to your cardio goal.

- Add resistance training for increased metabolic burn and tone. Resistance training is just as important as cardiovascular training.

- When doing resistance exercise, you have to burn it to earn it. The sensations of your muscles burning and the feeling of a little soreness afterwards are good signs that you are making positive changes.

- Resistance training will increase your metabolism and will keep your heart and body healthy.

- Do not obsess about sit-ups; instead, train your entire core.

- Exercise every day of the week.

- Exercise doesn't always have to be a "workout".

- Exercise as a family.

- Spend as much time outside as you can. We tend to stay inside too much.

- Always warm-up properly before doing anything physically demanding; five or ten minutes of light activity will suffice. Also, remember that the first ten minutes of exercise is always the hardest mentally, so push through and be kind to yourself during those minutes and you will find yourself enjoying your activities all the more.

- Flexibility is an essential part of health and fitness. The more limber your muscles are, the better your joints will respond and adapt to aging.

- Stretching helps elongate muscle structure as well as minimize post-exercise soreness. Be sure not to rush this important element of active living.

- Yoga and Tai Chi are incredibly rewarding practices to incorporate into your daily living. They develop the mind and body in ways no other exercise can.

- Rather than sending an email to a co-worker who is in your same building, walk to see them and deliver the message in person.

- Swim to get a full body, low-impact cardiovascular workout. If you don't know how to swim, it's never too late to learn this life-long sport. Sign up for lessons or stroke technique work with a coach so that you can increase your pool yardage for a longer, more enjoyable swimming experience.

- Hang out around those people who you define to be successful and they will be a positive influence on you. Also, surround yourself with people who are successful at incorporating exercise into their daily lives and you will find yourself doing the same.

- Start turning off the TV and internet more and remember that technology should never be the central component of our leisure.

ACTIVE CHALLENGES
FOR A SKINNY, SEXY MIND:

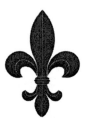

- Repeat the phrase "I *am* sexy" to yourself one hundred times in one day.

Do it and see how the power of what you tell your mind will transform you. *Remember, your body feeds on the thoughts you feed it.* Every aspect of your body language and body image depends upon the thoughts you allow your mind to think. This rule is without exception.

At the end of the day, write a journal entry describing the way you felt at the beginning of the day and then describe how you felt midday and at the end of the day. You may feel this is a silly exercise or that you will be lying to yourself. Go ahead, lie. You mind will eventually think it's the truth after enough repetition. *If you tell yourself that you are sexy, you will become sexy.*

- Have circumference measurements done by a friend or personal trainer and watch your body shrink and shape itself as you balance out your nutrition, cardio, and resistance exercise.

Keep track of your progress and as you are able to watch the numbers change you will find it much easier to prioritize fitness in your life. Everyone loves doing what they are good at, and everyone can be good at being fit.

Re-evaluate your progress on a monthly basis. Doing so will keep you accountable and motivated.

- Get three friends involved in exercise they don't normally do.

Do it and you will find out how inspiring your enthusiasm is to those around you. This challenge will keep you committed as you evangelize health and fitness to others. Your leadership in helping others along their path to health and *joie* will keep you focused on your own journey as well.

- Stop calling exercise a "workout" and start calling it "play-time" again.

The subconscious mind picks up on every negative statement we tell ourselves, and here, the word "work" can easily deter you from enjoying it. Remember the days of your childhood and how active you were when you played outside. Seek to mimic those days of movement and activity and you will begin looking forward to exercise.

- Start loving your body today instead of tomorrow and you will suddenly find that exercise becomes a lot easier.

Tomorrow may never come, and your beauty and body is not defined in a single dimension anyway. Beauty is multi-dimensional and if you start to love your body today, you will find that the world will be at your fingertips.

- Sign up for something active you have always wanted to do but never thought possible. Commit to it with another friend and start training a few months in advance.

Your mind is the only thing that limits you in life. Dream big and follow your dreams to fruition. Remember, nothing is impossible. If you need to lose two hundred pounds, you can do it. If you want to complete an Ironman but don't know how to swim yet, you can do it. If you want to change the world, you can do it.

Share your dreams with others and do not be afraid to vocalize them. The more you verbalize them out loud, the more your subconscious will commit to following through whole heartedly. Also, by sharing with others, you will have the support you need to help you through challenges and to celebrate with you in your victories.

- When you walk around doing your daily living activities, think about activating your muscles.

By doing so, you will start to be more aware of how your muscles move and will be able to consciously activate them throughout the day with better precision. It is easier to eat healthy and exercise when you appreciate the wondrous functions and workings of your body.

- Remember, strong is sexy.

You will continually grow in *joie* and beauty as you seek to fortify yourself emotionally, intellectually and physically. This type of strength takes a unique sense of self-awareness and analysis and it will serve you well in your ability to master your own *rhythm de vivre*.

- You are already beautiful. Embrace that and carry yourself accordingly with your newly mastered *skinny, sexy mind.*

LIVING ACTIVELY
Skinny, Sexy *à la carte*
On ne resiste pas l'invasion des idées.
[Don't resist new ideas.]

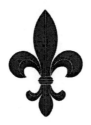

i. Skinny, Sexy SUMMARY:

"The fountain of youth is movement." -Mitch Thrower

ii. Skinny, Sexy REFLECTION:

Do you obsess or feel guilty about exercise, or is exercise an engrained part of your lifestyle? *How can you add five minutes extra physical activity to your daily live?* Taking the steps? Parking farther away? *Taking your dog for a longer walk?* Spending more time with your lover? *How much do you spend on gas for your car per month and how much could you save if you started bicycling locally?*

iii. Skinny, Sexy PERSONAL APPLICATION:

Experiment with moving your body. Try out three new types of "exercise" that are available to you and see what you most enjoy. Remember, the more you move, the younger you will look and feel and the more life you will be able to live. Try to stop calling it "exercise" and start thinking of it as "movement" and see how much better it feels. It feels good to move the body.

iv. Skinny, Sexy EATING:

Always make sure to eat within 45 minutes of completing a hard "workout"; your body is depleted after exercise and needs to be refueled in order to maximize the benefits of your workout and to maintain the integrity of your metabolism.

v. Skinny, Sexy YOU:

You *are* sexy. Commit to completing all of the active challenges for a skinny, sexy mind listed in this chapter. Love your body. Love yourself. Love life. Live life.

ABOUT THE AUTHOR

A natural born over-achiever, I have always expected perfection of myself. It is no wonder I bought into America's skinny revolution and subsequently battled an eating disorder in my quest for flawlessness.

I grew up in a loving middle-class family in the Lake of the Woods, VA, a private community in a rural area outside of Washington D.C. The youngest of two, I emulated the every move of my older brother and we developed a sibling rivalry that resulted in a dear, lifelong friendship.

I began swimming competitively when I was four, and my brother and I spent our childhood summers on the front porch swing dreaming of Olympic gold medals. My mother, a trained nurse, home-schooled the two of us so that we could continue to swim year-round at the level of competition we yearned for. By the time I was ten-years-old, I had set a United States National Age Group Record, meaning that I had the fastest time of any ten-year-old girl in American history in the 100-yard freestyle. I was nationally ranked in most events and had realistic expectations to make the Sydney Games.

My high school years were spent at Chatham Hall, an all-girls', college preparatory boarding school in southern Virginia that had an Olympic sized pool on campus. My father, a Union Pipefitter, worked a decade of overtime hours to finance my schooling. Puberty hit me at the same time that I hit a plateau athletically, and it was a recipe for disordered eating and a negative body image. I blamed my failure to be on track for my Olympic dream on my body and I began to hate food. My senior year in high school revolved around secret rendezvous to binge, laxative abuse, controlled calorie consumption, and six to seven hours of workouts a day; all the while I maintained an almost perfect G.P.A, took the maximum number of Advanced Placement classes, and was president of the student body.

My senior year, I was offered a coveted college scholarship to Davidson College in Charlotte, North Carolina. I accepted, and relished my four years of self-discovery there. My junior year, I did as any French major would and studied abroad. Tours, France introduced me to a world of tastes, fitness, and leisurely pace of life I never imagined possible. Living with a regionally renowned French chef who garnished my plate with a fattening affair of France's finest delicacies proved to be a nightmarish challenge that changed my life. My tastings in Tours awakened me to being kind to my body and sharpened my desire to compare the balance I felt so comfortably in France to my life in America.

After Davidson, I moved back to France as a full-time English teacher. I loved being integrated into the French educational system and getting an inside glimpse into the early development of French children. In my efforts to truly imitate French living, I did my best to emulate every aspect of the French. Oddly enough, in doing so, I developed a kinship with two other English speaking teachers, fondly referred to as the Trépied ("Tripod," *en français*) who transformed my understanding of *joie de vivre*. Together, on French soil, we discovered the ultimate secret to living not only comfortably, but joyfully in our own skins. The Trépied became legendary in Bordeaux, Périgueux, and even Paris; together, we learned to master the perfect Franco-American balance of sexiness, confidence and independence. We traveled Europe, playing hooky from work and becoming fine epicureans of every regional culinary specialty and connoisseurs of regional vintage wines.

I loved my body for the first time in my life in France; it was then that I knew my journey to freedom was lived and I needed to share it to help others. Please connect with me through my company Uncaged Confidence's various webpages (www.trishblackwell. com, www.beautifulbodybistro.com, www.uncagedconfidence. com, www.trainwithtrish.com), or on Twitter (@trainerTRISH) and join the community that believes in conquering life with confidence.

REFERENCES

Cash, Thomas F., Ph.D. *The Body Image Workbook: An 8-Step Program For Learning to Like Your Looks.* New Harbinger Publications, Inc. Oakland, CA. 1997.

Clarke, Stephen. *Talk to the Snail: Ten Commandments for Understanding the French.*_Boomsbury USA, New York, NY. 2006.

Huang, Al Chungliant and Jerry Lynch. *Thinking Body, Dancing Mind: TaoSports For Extraordinary Performance in Athletics, Business, and Life.* Bantam Publishing, US. June 1994.

Eldredge, John and Staci. *Captivating: Unveiling the Mystery of a Woman's Soul.* Thomas Nelson Publishing, July 2007.

Franklin, Regina. *Who Calls Me Beautiful? : Finding Our True Image in the Mirror of God.* Discovery House Publishing, Inc., Uhrichsville, OH. 2004.

Gibbs, Nancy. *The Magic of the Family Meal.* TIME Home page, 2006. TIME Magazine Online. January 15, 2010 http://www.time.com/time/magazine/article/0,9171,1200760,00.html

Katz, Nancy. *Eating Disorder Statistics*. Home page. 2000. United Health Foundation. September 19, 2004. http://womenissues.about.com/ls/eatingdisorders/a/edstats.htm

Long, Sarah. *Le Dossier, How to Survive the English.* John Murray Publishing, New York, January 2007.

Nadeau, Jean-Benoit and Julie Barlow. *Sixty Million Frenchmen Can't Be Wrong: Why We Love France But Not the French.* Sourcebooks, Naperville, Illinois, 2003.

National Association of Anorexia Nervosa and Associated Disorders, ANAD. Home page. April 2012. http://www.anad.org/get-information/about-eating-disorders/eating-disorders-statistics/

National Eating Disorders Association. Home page. April 2010. http://www.nationaleatingdisorders.org

Northwestern Health Sciences University. *Body Image Startling Facts.* Home page. April 2010. http://www.nwhealth.edu/healthyU/stayHealthy/eating2.html

Pollan, Michael. *Food Rules: An Eater's Manual.* Penguin Press, December 2009.

Omnivore's Dilemma: *A Natural History of Four Meals*, Penguin Press, London, 2006.

Roth, Geneen. *Breaking Free From Compulsive Eating.* Bobbs-Merrill Co., Inc. New York, NY.1986.

Centre National de Researche Scientique, le CNRS. Home page. March 2008. http://www.cnrs.fr

Williamson, Marianna. *A Return to Love: Reflections on the Principles of A Course in Miracles.* Harper Paperbacks, March 1996.

CPSIA information can be obtained at www.ICGtesting.com
Printed in the USA
BVOW07s2244131113

336211BV00002B/306/P